Ask the Grey Sisters

Sault Ste. Marie and the General Hospital, 1898-1998

Elizabeth A. Iles

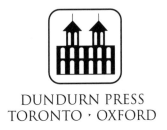

DUNDURN PRESS
TORONTO · OXFORD

Editor: Dennis Mills
Index: Claudia Willetts
Printer: Transcontinental Printing Inc.
Design: Cover: Telescope Graphic Design and Advertising   Text: Scott Reid
Front cover: Postcard showing the General Hospital, circa 1910. Courtesy Sault Ste. Marie Museum
Back cover: **Top:** Sault Ste. Marie at the turn of the century with the town's new General Hospital just visible at the top left. Hotel conveyances wait at the steamer dock to transport business people and tourists to the Cornwall, International, and other Sault hotels. Courtesy Sault Ste. Marie Museum. **Bottom:** The 1923 St. Mary's graduating class poses on the hospital's front steps. Dr. McRae (left) and Dr. Sinclair Sr. pose with Ethel Kennelly, Lesta Labelle, May Marshall, Genevieve McCann, Catherine McCarron, Winnifred McGee, and Noreen Owens. Courtesy Sault Ste. Marie General Hospital Inc. Archives.

Canadian Cataloguing in Publication Data

Iles, Elizabeth
     Ask the Grey Sisters: Sault Ste. Marie and the General Hospital, 1898-1998

Includes bibliographical references and index.
ISBN 1-55002-313-6

1. Sault Ste. Marie General Hospital — History.   I. Title.
RA983.S45S45 1998   362.1'1'09713132   C98-931493-6

1 2 3 4 5   02 01 00 99 98

We acknowledge the support of the **Canada Council for the Arts** for our publishing program. We also acknowledge the support of the **Ontario Arts Council** and the **Book Publishing Industry Development Program** of the **Department of Canadian Heritage.**

Printed and bound in Canada.

 Printed on recycled paper.

Dundurn Press   Dundurn Press   Dundurn Press
8 Market Street   73 Lime Walk   250 Sonwil Drive
Suite 200   Headington, Oxford   Buffalo, NY
Toronto, Ontario, Canada   England   U.S.A. 14225
M5E 1M6   OX3 7AD

Contents

To the General Hospital family

Grey Sisters past and present, physicians and staff members, auxilians and other donors of time, gifts, and talent, and to my own family

Doug, Michael, Johanna, and Peter

Sponsors' Foreword

A little more than one hundred years ago, Francis Clergue established four great industrial enterprises in Sault Ste. Marie.

Hydroelectric power generation came first, then transportation by rail and ship, pulp and paper manufacture, and finally, the production of steel.

The thriving community created by these industries needed a hospital to care for its growing citizenry and, in 1898, the General Hospital was born. For one hundred years, its story has been intertwined with the economic fortunes of Sault Ste. Marie.

Today, these four corporations are still the economic backbone of Sault Ste. Marie. As descendants of the original Clergue industries, we are proud of our long commitment to the people of this community and we proudly sponsor this centennial history of the Sault Ste. Marie General Hospital.

Algoma Steel Inc.   Algoma Central Corporation
Great Lakes Power Ltd.   St. Marys Paper Ltd.

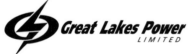

Foreword

For one hundred years, Grey Sisters have ministered to the people of Sault Ste. Marie and area through the sponsorship and ownership of the Sault Ste. Marie General Hospital.

Ask the Grey Sisters details the hospital's history and evolution over this one hundred years and will be a permanent record of what is achievable through dedication, collaboration and good will. We thank God for these wonderful years!

We are deeply grateful to all who have accompanied us over these years. They are many and the example of their dedication to serving the sick with love and compassion continues to this day and is an inspiratiion to all.

With hope and trust in Divine Providence, we move forward into the next century, seeking new ways to respond generously to the health needs of the Sault community.

May loving hearts and hands continue to be a powerful healing presence.

Sister Marguerite Hennessy

Sister Marguerite Hennessy
President Grey Sisters' Health System

When I visited the motherhouse of the Grey Sisters of the Immaculate Conception in Pembroke, I felt the presence of a spirituality that was deeply rooted in the Sisters' foundress, Saint Marguerite D'Youville.

In my association with the General Hospital, I have experienced that spirituality in action through the Sisters themselves, medical, nursing, administrative support staff and the many volunteers. Not only have they shared their many skills, they have given a part of themselves in living out their healing ministry.

As we continue to live through so many changes, may we draw strength from Saint Marguerite and all the men and women who have formed the General Hospital. It can be with a great deal of pride that we continue to strive to provide for the healthcare needs of our community and forge new partnerships with other healthcare providers, which will take us into the next one hundred years.

Mike Mingay

Mike Mingay
Chair Sault Ste. Marie General Hospital Board of Directors

Acknowledgements

First of all, thanks to Lois Krause, Rose Calibani, and Maggie Running, and to all of the Centennial committee members who have seen this project through as part of the centennial celebrations.

Thank you to many staff members, board members, and physicians, present and retired, who sat for interviews, answered questions, or read parts of the manuscript. A special thank you to two people: Manuela Giuliano, French language coordinator, who interpreted many of the French documents for me and provided the translation for the reminiscences of Sr. Ste. Constance; and to Mary Davies, pharmacist, who researched the 1926 pharmacy listing.

Thanks to many people from outside the hospital who also contributed their subject expertise: Linda Burtch, Willie Eisenbichler, Ken Griffith, Linda Kearns, Bill O'Donnell, Katherine Punch, and Chris Tossell in Sault Ste. Marie, and Jim Connor from the Hannah Institute in Toronto.

A special thank you to the Grey Sisters at the motherhouses in Pembroke and Ottawa for their very kind hospitality, especially to archivists Sr. Rita McGuire and Sr. Gertrude Harrington in Pembroke and Sr. Estelle Vaillancourt in Ottawa for their kindness and their expertise; also to Sr. Patricia Smith for details about Sr. St. Cyprien.

Finally, thanks to the staffs at the Sault Area Hospitals Library, Sault Ste. Marie Public Library, Wishart Library (Algoma University College), Sault Ste. Marie Museum, Metro Toronto Reference Library, Academy of Medicine Library (Bogusia Trojan and Sheila Swanson) and the Public Archives of Ontario for their expertise in preserving our history and making it available for study. Libraries and archives are an essential part of any society that wishes to celebrate and learn from its past.

Introduction
Ask the Grey Sisters

Ask the Grey Sisters

Sault Ste. Marie in the 1890s was a town in search of a hospital. As the town prepared to take its place in the 20th century, three powerful forces — from the business world, from medicine and from the community — all agreed that a community hospital was an essential centrepiece for a town with a future.

The businessman/industrialist was Francis H. Clergue, the larger-than-life American entrepreneur who was lured to Sault Ste. Marie by the hydroelectric potential of the rapids. Clergue and local Sault promoters like W.H. Plummer were attracting investors to the town with the promise of cheap, plentiful power. The Clergue industrial complex needed a community hospital to back it up.

The modern physician was Dr. Robert J. Gibson. Part of the vanguard of new "medical men" trained in Joseph Lister's method of aseptic surgery, Gibson knew that a hospital with professional nurses and a sterile operating room was a necessary part of the practice of modern medicine.

The new urban middle class was personified by Maria Plummer, the wife of one of the Sault's most prominent entrepreneurs, W.H. Plummer. Mrs. Plummer, her husband, and many others of like mind espoused the beliefs of the social gospel — that it was a citizen's social responsibility to ensure that neighbours were cared for in times of sickness.

How was the town to accomplish this monumental task, to create a hospital from nothing? The federal government turned down the town's request to fund a marine hospital as it had done in other port cities. Sir Oliver Mowat's provincial Liberal government felt little responsibility toward the sick of the province beyond paying for the institutional care of indigents. The municipal council felt that the town was on too shaky a financial basis to take on the burden of running a public institution. No citizens had as yet emerged who were wealthy enough to donate their home as a hospital. The town was at an impasse.

Then came a breakthrough. In June 1897, the provincial inspector of asylums and prisons, T.F. Chamberlain, came to town on his semi-annual tour of inspection. In the course of his stay, he met with the hospital committee. "If you wish a hospital of which the work is serious and lasting," he is reported to have told the committee, "ask the Grey Sisters." The rest, as they say, is history — and the subject of this book.

The Setting

By the shores of Gitchee Gumee
By the shining deep sea waters

Longfellow, *The Song of Hiawatha*

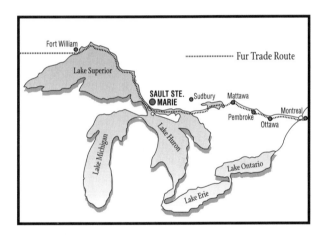

Sault Ste. Marie at the hub of the Great Lakes. The map shows the northern Ontario towns which had government-supported hospitals in 1900. All but the new boom town of Sudbury had roots in the fur trade.
Courtesy Telescope Graphic Design + Advertising

Sault Ste. Marie Hospital Core Values

Hospitality occurs when we behave in a kind and generous manner.

Hospitality
Spirituality
Vision
Justice
Sacredness of Life

The Community Beside the Rapids

The Community Beside the Rapids

From the aptly named Lake Superior, furthest inland and mightiest of the Great Lakes, to its more serene partner Lake Huron, the elevation drops approximately twenty feet over a distance of sixty-four miles. This descent is accomplished by a spectacular set of rapids along the upper course of the St. Mary's River. Père Dablon, one of the earliest of the Jesuit missionaries, described these rapids as a "violent current of waters from Lake Superior, which, finding themselves checked by a great number of rocks that dispute this passage, form a dangerous cascade half a league in width, all these waters descending and plunging headlong together, as if by a flight of stairs over the rocks which bar the whole river."

Sault Ste. Marie, the community beside the rapids, is one of the oldest settlements in North America. For at least 2,000 years, a parade of people has lived beside these jumping waters or "sault" of the St. Mary's River, and some of the greatest names of Canadian history — explorers, voyageurs, artists, soldiers, and traders — have portaged around and rested beside them.

The rapids provided an ideal environment for whitefish, and the archeological record suggests that for centuries a small community of Ojibwa lived close to the river, their livelihood based on whitefish. During summer months, the population swelled to the thousands as travellers from as far away as the upper Mississippi congregated to fish and trade for hides, tobacco, corn, maple sugar, and copper (from the sacred mines of Lake Superior). Bawating — the meeting place — was an apt name for this venerable settlement.

When the French came to North America in the 1600s and began to travel west, searching for furs and the elusive passage to the Orient, Bawating was a natural resting place. They called the natives there "les saulteurs," the people of the rapids, and they conferred and traded with the saulteurs while their huge "canots du maître" were being portaged around the rapids.

Étienne Brûlé, Champlain's protégé, was probably the first European to be seen by the Ojibwa at the Sault. He is reported to have travelled as far as the rapids while he explored the Mer Douce (Lake Huron) in 1618. Brûlé was followed in 1634 by Jean Nicolet, another agent for Champlain, who passed through the Sault du Gaston (newly named in honour of the brother of Louis XIII) in search of the passage to the Indies. Radisson and Groseilliers, on a reconnaissance mission for furs and in search of the same passage, arrived at the Sault in 1659 and called it a "terrestrial paradise." In 1668, Père Marquette established a Jesuit mission by the rapids, and the settlement took on its modern name, Sault Ste. Marie.

"The Sault" was considered so strategic to the French presence in North America that in 1671, when Sieur de St. Lusson, staged his elaborate pageant to claim all lands west of Montreal for the king, he chose to present it at Sault Ste. Marie.

St. Lusson was followed in 1731 by the great Canadian adventurer/explorer, Pierre de La Vérendrye, who travelled through Sault Ste. Marie on his search for the western sea. La Vérendrye was a giant in Canadian history, but readers of this story may have a greater interest in his nephew and expedition cartographer, Christophe Dufrost de Lajemmerais, brother to Marguerite d'Youville, foundress of the Grey Nuns. (Lajemmerais is profiled at the end of this chapter.)

The Pageant of St. Lusson notwithstanding, all French territory in North America passed into British hands following the Treaty of Paris in 1763, and the next great personage to travel to the Sault was the independent fur trader and explorer Alexander Henry in 1765.

By the turn of the century, Sault Ste. Marie was growing into a village of merchants, fur traders, farmers, and government officials. In 1812 Charles Oakes Ermatinger, fur trader, built his imposing stone residence beside the river, close to the government dock.

Throughout the 19th century, a string of the famous and not-so-famous passed through the village and rested there during their portage around the rapids. One group who would have caused little stir were four Grey Nuns who stopped over in the spring of 1844. Led by Sr. Marie-Louise Valade, they were enroute from the Grey Sisters' motherhouse in Montreal to establish a school at the Red River settlement on Lake Winnipeg. The four nuns made the trip by freighter canoe, passengers with a Hudson's Bay Company expedition on its way to the west. They had been given a personal send-off from Montreal by Hudson's Bay governor Sir George Simpson, and in the custom of the time, their heavy luggage had been sent by sea, travelling first to England, then back across the Atlantic to Hudson Bay, then by river to St. Boniface. Their trip, through the wind and storms of May, was anything but comfortable. "What can I say?" wrote Sr. Lagrave in a letter to her superior general, "I think the great gale over Lake Huron blows all my ideas away.... We have had bad weather nearly all the time and when the rain stops, the wind is nearly always against us. When we land to camp out, we are soaking with rain or shivering with cold. We make a good fire but we burn on one side and freeze on the other."

This little group would have been surprised to know that just fifty years later, two more Grey Sisters would make a comfortable one-day trip by train from Ottawa to Sault Ste. Marie to establish the new General Hospital.

As the 19th century wore on, Sault Ste. Marie increasingly became an isolated outpost. With the amalgamation of the Hudson's Bay Company and the North West Company in 1821, fur traders began to bypass the Sault for the more efficient northerly route, via Hudson Bay. In 1843 the Hudson's Bay Company finally closed its Sault post and the village's glory days of fur trading were over. In 1871, just after Confederation, the Sault's population stood at 880. By 1881 it had shrunk to 780.

Then suddenly, in the last decade of the old century, Sault Ste. Marie had a chance to enter the mainstream once more. And again, it was the presence of the rapids that brought the Sault to life. In 1890 the rapids were measured by Canadian engineer Alan Sullivan and were found to be hurling water toward Lake Huron at the tremendous rate of 125,000 cubic feet per second. The rapids, in other words, were rich in the commodity that every turn-of-the-century entrepreneur was searching for — "white coal," hydroelectric power.

Portrait

Christophe Dufrost de Lajemmerais

Christophe de Lajemmerais, youngest brother of Marguerite d'Youville, is an important historical figure in his own right, and interestingly enough, has his own connection with Sault Ste. Marie. Lajemmerais travelled through Sault Ste. Marie several times, little knowing that 160 years after his journeys a group of women religious, followers of his sister Marguerite, would arrive in the Sault to establish a hospital.

Lajemmerais's maternal uncle was Pierre de La Vérendrye, a giant in the annals of Canadian exploration. Christophe was a trusted second in command for several of his uncle's forays into the unknown west to discover the elusive western sea. He was also the expedition's cartographer and, according to the authoritative *Dictionary of Canadian Biography*, "[Christophe de Lajemmerais] has left us the first French map of the west, which is also the best." The map is dated 1733.

Born in December of 1708 at Varennes in New France, Christophe was the youngest of Marguerite's three brothers, being born just six months before their father died. Young Christophe entered the army in 1723 when he was 15 years old. There was lively interest at the time, both in New France and in the mother country, in discovering a passage to the great "Western Sea." At the time, prevailing thought held that the route lay along the Mississippi River. The discovery would be a scientific coup for France and would give the Canadians an upper hand over the British in establishing a fur-trading network.

In 1728, Lajemmerais's uncle, Pierre de La Vérendrye, took command of the poste du Nord, the land from Sault Ste. Marie to the north and west. By inquiring of the Indians who came to trade at the fort, La Vérendrye came to the correct belief: that the route to the west lay through the border lakes and that a fort on Lac Ouinipigon (Winnipeg) would be a key step forward in reaching the western sea.

In 1731 Lajemmerais joined his uncle's partnership and travelled on several expeditions from Quebec — first to Rainy River, then to Lake of the Woods, then to within a few kilometres of Lake Winnipeg. He died in May of 1736 at Fort Maurepas on the Red River and was buried near the present-day Manitoba village of Letellier.

Lajemmerais had made one return trip to Quebec in 1733 to confer with the expedition's financial backers and to inform the governor of their discoveries. At that time, his sister Marguerite was a newly widowed and financially destitute young woman, trying to care for her two young sons. Brother and sister would surely have met together to catch up on their news, and among their stories Christophe would have described for Marguerite the rapids at Sault Ste. Marie. Both would have been incredulous to learn of the hospital that would grow up close to those rapids and of the role that Marguerite would play in the story of that hospital.

Sault Ste. Marie in the 1890s

Sault Ste. Marie in the 1890s

The coming of the transcontinental railway after Confederation was a mixed blessing for Sault Ste. Marie. The CPR's main line bypassed the Sault completely, curving northwest from Sudbury through Biscotasing and Chapleau and on to the north shore of Lake Superior. However the 1887 completion of the Soo Line, the spur line from Sudbury to Sault Ste. Marie, led to a small employment boom and created a link with the Michigan rail system via the new International Railway Bridge. With the buoyancy created by this railway boom, Sault Ste. Marie incorporated as a town in 1887.

One year later, two of the Sault's greatest boosters, W.H. Plummer and James Conmee, headed up a consortium to construct a canal and harness the rapids for hydroelectric power. Their project failed spectacularly (one wall of the canal gave way when water was allowed in) but within ten years hydroelectric power, the new darling of modern entrepreneurs, would blast the Sault out of its provincial doldrums and into the industrial, urban 20th century. Sir Wilfrid Laurier's election cry, "the 20th century belongs to Canada!" could have been written with Sault Ste. Marie in mind.

Entrepreneurs on both sides of the river saw the potential of the rapids to attract industry and thus prosperity to the town. Their efforts attracted the attention of Francis H. Clergue, an extraordinary American entrepreneur, an archetypal "captain of industry" whose greatest weapon was "the overpowering salesmanship with which he disarmed potential investors of their doubts and instilled in them the profoundest confidence in both his own abilities and the merits of his schemes."[1]

Clergue burst on the Sault Ste. Marie scene in 1894 with his pockets filled with the money of Philadelphia coal and railway magnates. Boasting that he would change the rapids from "a health resort for the whitefish," Clergue took over Plummer's defunct Sault power company, secured $2,000,000 in backing from Philadelphia and incorporated the Lake Superior Power Company. Over the next five years, Clergue's eloquence parlayed this company into a sprawling network of industries, all dependent on power from the rapids. At its height in 1902, Consolidated Lake Superior encompassed power, pulp and paper, rail, and, most importantly, steel. The Helen Mine (named for a Clergue sister) at Michipicoten came into production in 1897 and in 1899 Clergue started the Algoma Central and Hudson Bay Railway (known

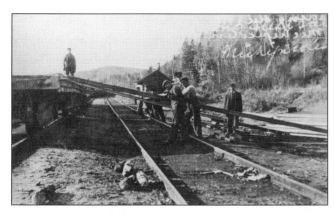

Francis Clergue mined the iron ore at Michipicoten, built a railway to carry the ore to his steel mill at Sault Ste. Marie, produced the power to run the mill, and manufactured steel rails from the ore. **Courtesy SSM Museum**

locally as "All Curves and High Bridges") to bring the ore to Sault Ste. Marie. The railway created a need for steel rails, and the Algoma Steel Corporation was chartered in 1901, rolling the first steel rails in Ontario in May 1902.

At the time, Clergue boasted that he employed 7,000 people and had a monthly payroll of $170,000. This same payroll would come back to haunt him only months later. In September 1903, failure to meet the payroll led to a riot, the entire Sault complex shut down, and Clergue was forced from power by Speyer & Co. of New York.

Clergue had failed to understand an obvious business truth: no company can survive without external customers, and his industries were an incestuous web of their own customers and providers. But Clergue had made one important and correct calculation. He understood that an industrial base in Sault Ste. Marie, steel in particular, dovetailed with the hopes and needs of all three levels of government — federal, provincial, and municipal. Sir Wilfrid Laurier in Ottawa was willing to ensure a Canadian steel industry by protecting Algoma Steel behind a $7 per rail tariff wall. George Ross's Liberals in Toronto were willing to guarantee Algoma's payroll in order to develop the Sault as the centre of "New Ontario," the undeveloped north which Toronto politicians expected soon to be filled with farmers and mining companies.

And finally, the town. Sault Ste. Marie, from the beginning, had embraced Clergue and his schemes as an elixir for local stagnation. Part of that elixir was the presence of a community hospital, both to serve as a centrepiece for the community, a signal to investors that this was a truly modern town, and also as a necessary civic institution to provide for the health needs of the workers and their families who were flocking to town.

A front-page spread "The Town of Sault Ste. Marie: A Brief Review of its Development and Progress ..." in the June 10, 1899 issue of the *Sault Express*, displays this understanding. Stating that the Sault "has shown more than ordinary enterprise in its efforts to attract investors and to encourage manufacturing industries," the article extolls the wonders of the power canal, the pulp mills, the healthful climate, the railway connection, the banking facilities, and, finally, the General Hospital. "Among the charitable institutions of the town," the writer asserts, "there is none so important as the new Hospital.... The building is a very imposing structure beautifully situated on the river bank in the eastern portion of the town.... It is complete and modern in all its appointments and visitors to this picturesque town will miss something if they fail to visit this handsome new hospital."[2]

The citizens of Sault Ste. Marie knew that the presence of a hospital was part of their ticket into the mainstream of the 20th century.

Portrait

Francis H. Clergue and the General Hospital

Francis H. Clergue is variously described as an ebullient, hard-selling American entrepreneur and a salesman and promoter whose grandiose schemes failed "with monstrous regularity." Nevertheless he was the dynamite that blasted Sault Ste. Marie into the industrial 20th century. Sir James Dunn had the kindest description of Clergue, saying, "Mr. Clergue just willed that a wilderness should become an industrial community. [He] laid it out on a broad and generous scale and the chinks are gradually being filled in."[3]

Clergue's relationship with the General Hospital conveys yet another facet of the Clergue mystique — a man of great personal charm and gallantry who had a naive delight in giving gifts. A newspaper account of the inauguration of a new hospital elevator and a "state of the union" letter from the first hospital administrator, Sr. Marie du Sauveur, to her superior general both contain charming Clergue vignettes.

In January of 1900 Clergue and one of his sisters paid a New Year's visit to the newly opened hospital and, as a New Year's gift, offered to purchase an elevator and to provide the power for it "so long as the hospital exists." "I consider the General Hospital the most important public institution possible to establish," he wrote to Dr. Gibson after the visit, "and I am glad to let you know of my agreeable surprise in finding the Institution so well laid out and equipped.... The Architectural appearance of the building is disappointing but that can be improved at any time."[4]

Clergue and an associate from Montreal, George Drummond (governor of Montreal's Royal Victoria Hospital and brother to Sault physician Dr. Drummond) were in attendance for the elevator's "inaugural hoist," as were Drs. Gibson, Reid, McCaig, Flemming, and McLean, Crown Attorney Kehoe, MPP C.N. Smith, and Mayor Plummer.

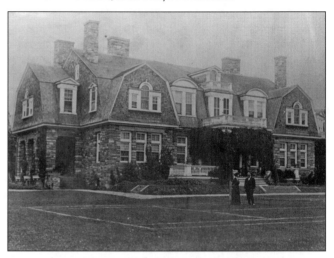

Clergue's beautiful home Montfermier, with Clergue and probably a sister on the tennis court. The house overlooked the town from Mofley Hill. In 1926, after Clergue's death, a series of letters passed between his executors and the Grey Sisters regarding purchase of the magnificent estate for a college.
Courtesy SSM Museum

Clergue and Sr. Marie du Sauveur made the first trip in the elevator. Then

> when the entire party had been elevated to the top floor of the building they were introduced to a decanter of homemade cordial ... and a table of delicacies which had been elaborately spread by the sisters. The hospital's staunchest friend, Dr. Gibson, sat at the head of the board and acted as toastmaster.... Mr. Clergue's health was drunk with much enthusiasm and in acknowledging the

compliment he made a splendid speech. One of the thoughts which he gave expression to was that it ought to be impossible for human suffering to exist if it is possible for human skill to prevent it. A deep sympathy for his fellow beings who were afflicted by ailments of body or mind was a part of his nature and he could not get away from it if he would. To be able, even though in a small way to assist in the alleviation of suffering humanity was a source of much satisfaction to him and he desired to state that as there was a pressing need for an isolation hospital in Sault Ste. Marie he would gladly subscribe $500 toward the cost of such a building provided however the town did its full duty in the matter.... The evening throughout was most enjoyably spent by all present, everybody was toasted and many felicitous speeches were made and as the hour hand pointed close to 12 the party sang "God Save the Queen" and went home.[5]

Later that year Sr. Marie du Sauveur wrote to her Superior General:

To my honourable Mother Kirby ... Monday morning, at around 9:00, Mr. F.H. Clergue arrived at the hospital with three VIPs [gros monsieurs]. He asked me if it was too early in the morning to visit the house [the hospital]. I answered that he should feel free to come at any time. Upon entering the kitchen, he remarked that the stove was too small and offered to replace it with a bigger one. Naturally I accepted because the stove really is too small.

He seems proud of the hospital. He brought the men everywhere, pointing out the beauty of the gardens. On their return to the visiting room, I offered them a small glass of Benedictine, which they accepted with pleasure. We drank the Benedictine, toasting the prosperity of the house.[6]

Two years later, Clergue's entire Sault empire began to unravel. With few external customers for its products and, hobbled by unwisely choosing Bessemer steel production over open hearth, the company closed down its steel works and the corporation went into bankruptcy. Clergue was no longer "the Sault's great captain of industry," but the enterprises he forced into being — transportation, steel, power, and paper — still form the industrial backbone of Sault Ste. Marie today, and the hospital, which he in large part brought into being, continues to care for its citizens.

Health and Medicine in the Late 19th Century

Health and Medicine in the Late 19th Century

The half century from 1870 to 1920 was a period of revolutionary change for health care and for hospitals in Ontario. It was an era that saw the "transformation of the hospital from a Victorian secular charity for the indigent and working poor into a workplace for the production of health for all members of the community."[7] A 1934 survey of hospitals stated, "Less than a generation ago, our public hospitals existed solely as public charities for the care of the indigent sick in our midst. Today all classes of people of this Province are on the whole, admirably and adequately served."[8]

After 1920, hospital changes can be seen as refinements and advancements — the basic shape and form of modern medicine and the modern hospital were already in place. A hospital patient of 1920 would understand the hospital of the 1990s, even though most of the equipment would be a cause for wonder. But a mid-19th century Ontario resident would not have been able to imagine the hospital experience of the early 20th century, so profound were the changes.

Until the modern hospital began to take shape, there was little incentive, aside from some surgical procedures, for members of the middle class to enter a hospital. American historian Charles Rosenberg observes that at mid-1800s, "The middle class home with its clean environment, domestic servants, familial care and private physician was a preferable milieu for the convalescent." Hospitals were few and far between and they were only of value for those who were without a source of nursing care. Those with a family or the ability to hire a nurse had little need for a hospital.

But as the 20th century neared, changes in the practice of medicine made the services of a hospital more necessary. Surgical anaesthesia using ether was introduced at mid-century and was widely used within several years. Joseph Lister's germ theory swept North America from 1870 onward, and the elite of Canadian surgeons travelled to Lister's home territory in Britain for postgraduate training. No longer could surgeons wipe their scalpels on their jackets or rest the scalpel by holding it between their teeth. No longer would they walk from the autopsy room to the operating theatre wearing the same jacket and without washing their hands. The stethoscope and thermometer came to be used as more than curiosities and the patient's temperature was charted and studied. X-rays were introduced to Canadian hospitals in the 1890s. The hospital laboratory began to give valuable information from some rudimentary blood and urine tests. The notion of specific diseases became more common, and physicians began to approach disease by empirical investigation — investigations that often used equipment that could only be found in a hospital.

At the same time, the administrative and nursing methods popularized by Florence Nightingale were changing hospital administrators and nurses into professionals. And finally, no longer was the surgeon's major expense the purchase of his set of surgical instruments. Now surgery could only be performed in the controlled atmosphere of a hospital operating room where the assistants were professional nurses; the equipment, linens, and instruments were sterile; the surgeon wore rubber gloves (invented in 1890) and a gown; and the operation was conducted in a haze of carbolic mist. The hospital operating room became "the most plausible and convenient place to perform surgery. To many surgeons in fact, it was beginning to seem the only ethical place to practice an increasingly demanding art."[9]

An indication of just how much surgery had captured the popular imagination can be gleaned from Ralph Connor's popular 1906 novel *The Doctor: A Tale of the Rockies.* "I'll take you to see my cases," thunders the old physician to the young man who has come to him to seek an apprenticeship, "and by God's help, we'll make you a surgeon! A surgeon, sir! You've got the fingers and the nerves. A surgeon! That's the only thing worth while. The physician can't see further below the skin than anyone else. He guesses and experiments, treats symptoms, trys one drug then another, guessing and experimenting all along the line. But the knife, boy!... There's no guess in the knife point!"[10]

The doctor goes on to pinpoint the exact difference between the older form of medicine, which treated symptoms and modern medicine, which investigates in order to make a diagnosis and then treats accordingly. "Look at that boy Kane, died three weeks ago," the doctor counsels his young apprentice. "'Inflammation,' said the physician. Treated his symptoms properly enough. The boy died. At the postmortem ... the knife discovered an abscess on the vermiform appendix ... I believe in my soul that the knife at the proper moment might have saved that boy's life!"[11]

By the 1890s, hospitals had become essential to the effective practice of medicine in Ontario.

But if modern medicine and modern hospitals had arrived, the legislation to deliver them adequately to the citizens of Ontario most assuredly had not arrived with them. The British North America Act of 1867 had given the federal government responsibility for quarantine, marine hospitals, and health services for natives and the armed forces. In other words, the federal government took responsibility for services that were expected to be expensive, including disease control and treatment.

The provinces were given responsibility for "the establishment, maintenance and management of hospitals, asylums and charities ... other than marine hospitals," in other words, the regulation of institutions that housed those who could not care for themselves — orphans, indigents who were sick or elderly, the mentally ill, and those in prison. The Charity Aid Act of 1874 set out the extent of the Ontario government's understanding and support of hospitals. The newly created inspector of prisons, asylums and public charities was to make a yearly inspection of all such institutions, thus making them eligible for grants. Support to hospitals was set at a daily grant of twenty cents per patient, a rate that rose with each amendment to the Act.

Finally the Hospitals and Charitable Institutions Act of 1897 established grants for patients who did not pay more than $7.00 per week, thus differentiating for the first time between paying and indigent patients and also effectively capping the weekly hospital rate for most patients at $7.00. (Hospitals were thus able to collect from the patient and from the government.) This legislation was amended several times, upping the provincial stipend and enunciating the municipalities' contribution, and finally in 1931, it was renamed the Public Hospitals Act.

The provincial government disassociated itself from "health" (i.e. public health) with the passage of the Public Health Act of 1884, which made health a municipal responsibility. Municipalities were to create boards of health and hire sanitary inspectors.

Legislative support and funding for hospitals were thus fragmented, informal, and haphazard. Control was divided among the three levels of government — "Ottawa," the province, and municipality — the latter two giving a parsimonious grant, with paying patients expected to take up the slack. No level of government was willing to take on the expense and effort of controlling and funding this peculiar new institution. Like Topsy, the modern hospital in Ontario had "just growed."

Portrait

Typhoid, Diphtheria, Scarlet Fever, Smallpox ...

Infectious diseases were the scourge of northern Ontario in the late 1900s and early decades of the 20th century. Today they are almost unheard of — smallpox has even been stamped out — but a little more than 100 years ago, names such as typhoid and diphtheria struck terror in the settlements of the north.

Waves of people poured into and through Algoma around the turn of the century. Lumber camps sprang up along the north shore of Lakes Huron and Superior to harvest the red and white pine, spruce, and balsam. Minerals were prospected for and mined — copper at Bruce Mines, and iron ore at Michipicoten. The new canal at Sault Ste. Marie brought in hordes of construction workers and then allowed travellers by the hundreds to pass through town on their way to Lake Superior and the west.

With this movement of people came disease. Living quarters in the camps were crowded, sanitation was primitive, pasteurization was non-existent, and there was little understanding of the crucial importance of a safe water supply.

The federal government's response to the threat of epidemics was to establish and fund marine hospitals at the most vulnerable points, port cities. The municipal response to individual outbreaks was to commandeer any available building for quarantining unfortunate victims. Depending on the finances of the community, these institutions were called isolation hospitals, sheds, or tents, and generally they were outfitted starkly and primitively.

But it was the provincial government through its mandating and control of municipal Boards of Health which finally won the battle against infectious disease. Sewers, a regulated water supply, vaccination programs, enforced pasteurization of milk, and chlorination of municipal water supplies finally took the terror out of these diseases and relegated them to the history books.

Typhoid outbreaks in Sault Ste. Marie, especially among steamer passengers and lumber camp workers, were among several factors that led to the opening of the General Hospital. Many of the hospital's patients in the early years were typhoid victims.

The Grey Sisters

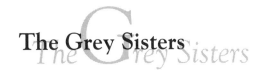

I leave all to Divine Providence.
All will happen which is pleasing to God.

Marguerite d'Youville

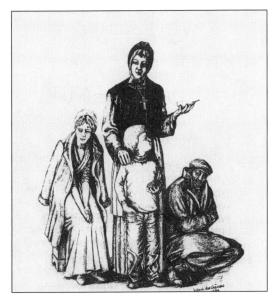

Marguerite d'Youville
Courtesy Sisters of Charity of Montreal

Sault Ste. Marie Hospital Core Values

Spirituality is our commitment to providing an atmosphere where any person who enters our hospital will receive reverence and respect.

Hospitality

Spirituality

Vision

Justice

Sacredness of Life

The Catholic Tradition in Healthcare

When the town of Sault Ste. Marie was searching for an organization that could rise to the challenge of building and maintaining a hospital, they quite naturally turned to the Catholic Church — an institution that for centuries had maintained hospital refuges for society's unfortunates. To appreciate the story of the General Hospital, it is necessary to understand the two orders of Grey Sisters who have owned the hospital and the woman who is the spiritual foundress for these orders. The inspiration for both orders was Marguerite d'Youville, a remarkable woman who was born in New France in 1701.

Hospitals, refuges of hospitality for strangers, have been a part of every civilization — from the state-mandated hospitals of Asoka, emperor of India, to the nosocomia of Rome. During the late Middle Ages, hospitals emerged across France to extend hospitality to travellers and pilgrims and others who could not care for themselves — the destitute, the elderly, and the orphaned. Some were guided by orders of monks (notably the ancient Knights Hospitallers), but as the concept of hospitals flourished, new religious orders (mainly female) dedicated to nursing sprang up to maintain them.

When the French crossed the Atlantic in the 1600s to set up their colonies in New France, the nursing sisters, notably the Sisters of the Misericord and the Ursuline Nuns, came to minister to the settlers. Along with them came the concept of hospital refuges for the destitute and the sick.

The religious orders founded two types of hospitals in New France, the hôtel-dieu (literally the hostel of God) and the general hospital. The hôtels-dieu were akin to modern hospitals in that they ministered to the sick. Their mission was to allow the sick person a time of grace and respite for moral and physical regeneration. The Hôtel-Dieu in Quebec City, founded by the Misericords in 1639, was the first hospital in Canada. Montreal's Hôtel-Dieu was founded by Jeanne Mance in 1644. The general hospital had a broader mission: it was designed as a refuge for those who could not care for themselves for reasons of age, poverty, or circumstance, as well as sickness. General hospitals cared for the aged, the disabled, and mentally ill, for abandoned children, prostitutes, and "fallen" women. In Montreal, the General Hospital was founded in 1692 by the Freres Charron. In 1747, ownership of the hospital was given to Marguerite d'Youville and her new order of Grey Sisters.

In 1820 construction began on Toronto General, cited as the first hospital in Upper Canada. Interestingly though, several histories state that the honour of earliest hospital in Upper Canada should go to Sault Ste. Marie, where a small hospital was established by the Jesuits as part of their mission to the Ojibwa.

For the sisters in these institutions, ministering to the needs of the sick and the destitute was seen as a way of serving God. These women were truly living Jesus' words, "Inasmuch as you have done it to the least of these my brethren, you have done it unto me." The most famous of the modern nursing nuns voiced this same belief. "I see God in every human being," wrote Mother Teresa. "When I wash the leper's wounds I feel I'm nursing the Lord himself. Is it not a beautiful experience?"

When the town of Sault Ste. Marie approached the Grey Sisters of the Cross to establish a hospital, this is the ancient tradition that was being continued. Time and again, the reminiscences of the early sisters in Sault Ste. Marie describe seeing the face of Jesus in their patients. The hardships the sisters endured, which were many, were bearable for the mission they were accomplishing. As a child, their foundress and inspiration, Marguerite d'Youville, had been educated by the Ursuline Nuns, the most prominent nursing order in New France. As an adult, and as the administrator of the Montreal General Hospital, Marguerite said to her small band of followers, "the people must know that we never refuse to serve."

Marguerite d'Youville, Foundress of the Grey Sisters

Marguerite Dufrost de Lajemmerais, foundress of the Grey Sisters, belonged to one of the great families of New France. She was born October 15, 1701, the eldest child of François-Christophe Dufrost de La Gemerais and Marie-Renée Gaultier de Varennes. La Gemerais was a career military officer who had ably served Governor Frontenac at the garrisons at Niagara and Cataraqui (Kingston). His wife was the daughter of René Gaultier, governor of Trois Rivières.

Marguerite, the eldest of six children, grew up in her grandfather's seigneury at Varennes, about twenty miles from Montreal. Six months before the birth of the sixth child, Captain La Gemerais died unexpectedly, throwing his family into great financial hardship. The child, named Christophe in memory of his father, grew up to become a famous Canadian in his own right. He has his own interesting connection with Sault Ste. Marie, described earlier in this book.

At the age of 11, Marguerite was sent for two years to be schooled at the Ursuline Convent in Quebec City. At 21, she married François-Madeleine d'Youville, a wealthy and handsome young man who was part of the entourage of the governor of Montreal. Her married life had all the elements of a domestic tragedy: an overbearing and unsympathetic mother-in-law, difficulties with money, and a husband who involved himself with the illicit and disreputable trade in liquor with the natives. Added to this were Marguerite's sorrows as a mother — four of her six children died in infancy.

D'Youville himself died in 1730, leaving Marguerite at age 28 with two small sons, a mountain of debt, and the public infamy of her late husband's involvement in illegal activities. In her suffering, Marguerite began to take solace in the church. But at the same time, she took practical steps to provide a decent life for herself, her sons, and, finally, for the destitute that she saw around her. Practical good sense, a feeling of mission toward the poor, a belief in the hand of God, and a great joy in life became the touchstones of her life. Immediately following her husband's death, Marguerite set to organizing a small shop in her home in the Place du Marche to provide for herself and her children. She devoted her life to God as a member of the Confraternity of the Holy Family at Notre Dame Church and began to regularly visit the lonely and destitute who inhabited the old, dilapidated Montreal General Hospital.

By 1737 Marguerite had resolved to spend her life

serving the poor, the imprisoned, and the sick, certain in the feeling that in serving the poor, she was serving Christ himself. A small group of like-minded women joined with her and together they moved into a large stone house on Notre Dame Street. This event is now considered to mark the founding of her religious order. "We are the servants of all for the sake of the poor," she told her companions, "and everyone must know that we never refuse to serve."

The early years were filled with setbacks — they were openly taunted and jeered as les soeurs grises (the tipsy nuns) an allusion to François d'Youville's association with the liquor trade. Finally, in 1747, Marguerite and her companions were given control of the aging Montreal General Hospital, a once-great institution which they brought back to life. One of her first actions was to open the hospital to female patients as well as to men, and by opening the hospital to victims of a smallpox epidemic, she transformed it from a hospice into a true hospital.

In 1753, the group received official designation as a religious order, officially known as the Sisters of Charity of the General Hospital, but commonly and affectionately known as Les Soeurs Grises, the Grey Nuns (Sisters).

Marguerite's last years were as difficult as the early ones — the fall of Montreal in 1760 and the ceding of New France to the British, the return to France of many of her family members after the conquest, and a disastrous fire that destroyed their hospital in 1765. "My dear Father," Marguerite wrote to her spiritual advisor, "pray that God will give me the strength to bear all these crosses and to make saintly use of them. So much at one time: to lose one's king, one's country, one's possessions, one's friends."

Despite these hardships, Marguerite continued her good works until her death in 1771 at the age of 70. The *Dictionary of Canadian Biography* praises her remarkable administrative talent, her unselfishness, and her indomitable courage but stresses that these, "should not obscure the sensitivity of this woman, who was moved by the misfortunes as well as by the moments of happiness of her relatives and friends and whom every form of human affliction touched deeply." In the 200 years since her death, Marguerite's life and beliefs have inspired Grey Sisters working from six autonomous motherhouses: in Montreal, Ste. Hyacinthe, Quebec City, Ottawa, Pembroke, and Philadelphia. She was canonized in 1990 — the first Canadian-born saint and truly a saint for our times — a poor, single mother from Montreal.

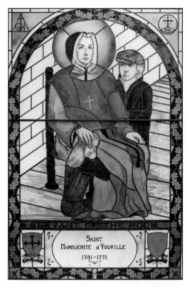

Marguerite's name is remembered at the General Hospital by a hospital wing, a street which skirts the hospital grounds, and a small park between the hospital and the St. Mary's River. This stained-glass donor board was commissioned by the hospital's Foundation at the time of her canonization in 1990. Designed and crafted by local artist John Hawke, it stands in the hospital's main lobby.

The Sisters of Charity and the Grey Sisters of the Immaculate Conception

The present owners of the General Hospital are the Grey Sisters of the Immaculate Conception, based in Pembroke. But it was neither they nor the original Grey Sisters from Montreal who were the hospital's foundresses. Rather, that honour belongs to a third group, the Sisters of Charity of Ottawa (Grey Sisters of the Cross).

At her death in 1771, Marguerite d'Youville left behind a strong and committed group of followers, and the Sisters of Charity of Montreal — Les Soeurs Grises — grew and prospered. In 1840 four sisters travelled to Ste. Hyacinthe to establish a hospital, and in 1844 another small group (discussed earlier in this book) journeyed to the Red River settlement to teach.

At the same time, the now-British colony of Quebec was growing and prospering. In 1791, following the American revolutionary war and the influx of the Loyalists, the colony was divided along the Ottawa River into two provinces, Upper and Lower Canada. During the 1800s, the Ottawa valley was heavily settled by Irish and Scottish immigrants, who cleared farms and started up a thriving lumber industry. Bytown (later renamed Ottawa) grew up where the Rideau and Ottawa rivers met.

In 1844 Bishop Phelan of Kingston petitioned the Grey Sisters to come to Bytown to teach the French and Irish Catholic girls of the Ottawa valley. Sister Elisabeth Bruyère, 26 years old at the time, was to lead the group. "Go, daughters of the cross," said the Bishop of Montreal, giving his blessing to them and at the same time bestowing on them the name by which they would become popularly known — the Grey Sisters of the Cross.

The Bytown group of Grey Sisters was meant to be governed from Montreal but the journey across a provincial boundary made that difficult, and in 1851 the Ottawa sisters were given their independence so that they could more easily follow the laws of Ontario in their schools. Mother Elisabeth Bruyère thus became their foundress, and their motherhouse still stands where it was built in 1850, at 9 Bruyère Street, close to Sussex Drive. In 1968 they reaffirmed their official name, the Sisters of Charity of Ottawa.

As the 19th century moved on, the Ottawa Grey Sisters carried on their mission with zeal. Their numbers grew to almost 450 by the turn of the century with many of the novices being daughters of the Irish settlers from up and down the Ottawa valley (thus the Irish flavour and lilt to many celebrations over the years at our General Hospital in Sault Ste. Marie).

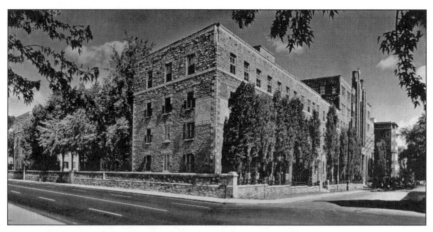

The motherhouse of the Sisters of Charity of Ottawa, standing just around the corner from the Parliament Buildings. The decision was made here to send four sisters to found a hospital in far-off Sault Ste. Marie.   **Malak photo. Courtesy SCO**

They established places of refuge for society's unfortunates in Ottawa and many schools and convents on both sides of the Ontario–Quebec border. Ottawa General was their first hospital, opened in 1866, and in 1878, they opened Mattawa General and Pembroke General. In Mattawa, the original building, startlingly similar to the first General Hospital in Sault Ste. Marie, still stands with its commanding view of both the Ottawa and Mattawa Rivers. By 1898 the Ottawa Congregation (Grey Sisters of the Cross) owned a total of six hospitals in Ontario, Quebec, and New York.

In 1896 they had established St. Joseph's Hospital in the new nickel-and-railway boom-town of Sudbury, taking over a tiny hospital that had been established by the Canadian Pacific Railway. One of the four sisters sent to work in Sudbury was Sr. St. Cyprien, who was to play a crucial role in influencing her order to come to Sault Ste. Marie in 1898. "Everyone here," she wrote to Superior General Demers in 1897 from Sudbury, "says the Sault is the place of the future."

The work of the Grey Sisters of the Cross was also known to another notable person, T.F. Chamberlain, inspector of prisons and asylums for the province of Ontario, who counselled the Sault's hospital committee, "If you wish a hospital of which the work is serious and lasting, ask the Grey Sisters."

Mère Demers's term as superior general ended in 1897, just after the sisters were approached by the people of the Sault, and she was replaced by Superior General Dorothy Kirby. Mère Kirby was born at Fitzroy Harbour, close to Ottawa, the daughter of Irish immigrant parents. She was 57 at the time of her appointment, and her ten-year tenure was a time of continued expansion for the Grey Sisters of the Cross, both in Canada and the northern U.S. As well as the hospital in Sault Ste. Marie, the Grey Sisters founded hospitals in Maniwaki and Buckingham, Quebec, and in Ogdensburg and Plattsburg, New York, during Mère Kirby's time of office.

If provincial boundaries were the cause of the separation between the Grey Sisters in Montreal and

Ottawa, it was difficulties of language within the Ottawa congregation that led to the creation in the 1920s of two new English-speaking orders from the Grey Nuns of the Cross. In 1926, the General Hospital in Sault Ste. Marie was given to one of these newly created orders, the Grey Sisters of the Immaculate Conception .

Through the early years of the 20th century, the Grey Sisters of the Cross were the only bilingual community of sisters to have their motherhouse in the Ottawa area. As a result, many of the Irish-Catholic girls from the area entered the order. As they also opened schools, convents, and hospitals in several American northeastern states, many more English-speaking girls came to admire the order and decided to enter. By 1920 almost one quarter of the novices that had been received into the order were English speaking (643 French and 199 English).

A reorganization was inevitable, and the first split came in 1921 when 155 American English-speaking Grey Sisters were permitted to form their own congregation. They became the Grey Nuns of the Sacred Heart with their motherhouse located in Philadelphia. This left the Canadian English-speaking Greys concerned about their future and worried that English-speaking novices were choosing other orders. So they, too, petitioned the Vatican to allow them to create an autonomous congregation. Finally, in 1926, a letter arrived from the Vatican stating that,

> the English-speaking Religious who so request should be separated from the ... Ottawa Institute of the Sisters of Charity of the Cross and should form a new Pontifical Congregation ...The Mother-House and Novitiate of the new Congregation should be established within the limits of the diocese of Pembroke ... The Convent existing in Pembroke Town shall ...become the property of the new Institute, as likewise the Hospital in the City of Sault-Sainte-Marie but with the obligation upon the new Congregation of paying the debts that are upon the Hospital itself. But the Mattawa Hospital shall remain the property of the Ottawa Institute.[12]

The mortgage on the Sault hospital was stated to be $98,000 with $73,000 owing to the motherhouse and $25,000 to external creditors.

The new order was duly formed. Sister St. Paul became the first superior general, governing a community of seventy-seven sisters, with their motherhouse established in Pembroke. As well as the hospital in Sault Ste. Marie, they were given the school and hospital in Pembroke, the Eganville convent and the St. Patrick Orphanage in Ottawa. They took the name Grey Sisters of the Immaculate Conception and the motto "to Jesus through Mary." Twenty-four postulants entered the new order in its first year.

Far away at the hospital in Sault Ste. Marie, the news was a shock. Sisters who had devoted close to

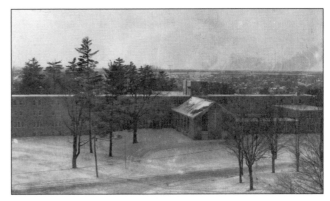

The motherhouse of the Grey Sisters of the Immaculate Conception in Pembroke. The building overlooks the historic Ottawa River.
Courtesy GSIC

thirty years of service to the people of the Sault would have to leave and new sisters from a struggling new order would have to come and pick up the reins. It was a bittersweet time for the young hospital and the town. Sister Ste. Constance who had been at the hospital almost from the beginning, wrote in her memoirs, "I will not speak of the scene of our departure; there would be too many sad things to say."

A new chapter began in the life of the General Hospital and a new relationship which has continued and prospered for seventy years. As well as the hospitals in Sault Ste. Marie and Pembroke, the Grey Sisters of the Immaculate Conception have gone on to administer hospitals in Lestock, Saskatchewan (St. Joseph's Hospital, 1937–1981), Esterhazy, Saskatchewan (St. Anthony's Hospital, 1940–1989) and Penetanguishene, Ontario (Penetanguishene General, from 1942).

In the summer of 1997, exactly 250 years after Marguerite d'Youville took on the work of the destitute at Montreal General Hospital, representatives of all six orders of Grey Sisters gathered in Buffalo to celebrate their common heritage. One of the presenters, Sr. Marie Bonin from Montreal, traced the amazing growth of the orders and their spread around the world. She concluded her presentation by saying, "This humble woman, Marguerite d'Youville founded our congregation. This humble woman influenced the world with her charism."

Grey Sisters Today

Six independent orders of Grey Sisters are at work today. All have evolved from the original Sisters of Charity of Montreal, and all look to Marguerite d'Youville as their foundress.

1753   Sisters of Charity of Montreal
        (Mère Marguerite d'Youville)

1840   Sisters of Charity of Ste. Hyacinthe
        (Mère Archange Thuot)

1849   Sisters of Charity of Quebec
        (Mère Marcelle Mallet)

1851   Sisters of Charity of Ottawa
        (Mère Elisabeth Bruyère)

1886   Sisters of Charity of the Hôtel-Dieu of
        Nicolet (joined with Sisters of Charity of
        Montreal in 1941)

1921   Grey Nuns of the Sacred Heart, Philadelphia
        (Mother Mary Augustine)

1926   Grey Sisters of the Immaculate Conception,
        Pembroke (Mother St. Paul)

Portrait

The Chapel

The old chapel and hospital are gone but their memories live on with many people, and parts of the chapel itself live on, both in the present hospital chapel and in other sanctuaries in Pembroke and at Goulais River.

The first mass in the hospital chapel was celebrated just weeks after the sisters had moved into the new building on Queen Street. It was August 15, 1898, the Feast of the Assumption, and the mass was celebrated by Fr. Carré from Sacred Heart. The priest brought his own altar items and the sisters added several vases of wildflowers. "In spite of our poverty," notes the *Chronicles*, "the little chapel took on a festive air and we felt happy to possess under our roof the Divine

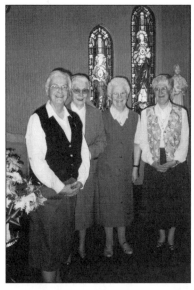

Srs. Marguerite Hennessy, Macrina, Margaret Holt, and Madeline Cooke, all previous General Hospital employees, in the chapel in Pembroke. Behind them are the windows from the old chapel.

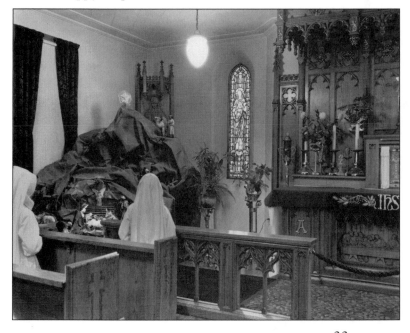

The chapel in the old hospital, decorated for Christmas. The carved front of the altar was kept and is mounted on one wall of the new chapel. The stained glass windows are in Pembroke. Note the shamrocks framing the window. The sisters are most likely nurses since they are wearing white.

Host. We hope that the good Lord will bless the works of his daughters."[13]

When the old hospital was demolished, parts of the chapel were given to other sites. The pews were installed in the balcony of the new chapel and two of the stained-glass windows were installed in the sisters' private chapel on the B Wing, fourth floor. In 1989, when that floor was no longer used as a residence, the chapel was dismantled and the windows were sent to Pembroke where they now grace the chapel at Shalom, the sisters' long-term-care residence. The altar was sent to the church at Goulais River, all except the frieze of the Last Supper from the altar's face. The frieze was kept as a memento and is mounted on the back wall of the present hospital chapel.

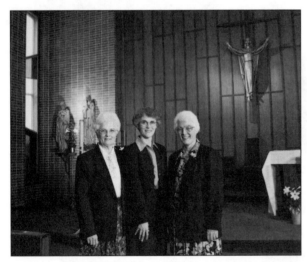

Srs. Jean Grey, Mary Buckley, and Diane Carty are the Grey Sisters currently working at the hospital. They are pictured in the chapel. Sr. Madeline Cooke is absent from the photo.

The Hospital

Viewing the magnificent structure fronting on Queen Street
with its beautiful lawns and village of buildings, sheds …
we can hardly believe that ten years ago we had no hospital at all.

The Sault Star, June 11, 1908

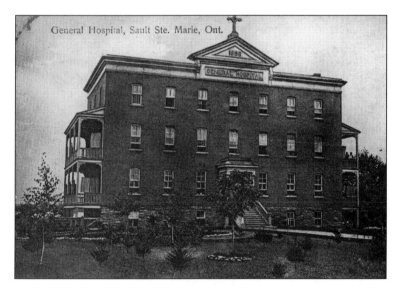

A postcard of the first hospital building on Queen Street, with its beautiful
sun porches and imposing roofline.

Sault Ste. Marie Hospital Core Values

Vision is our ability to anticipate, plan, and make provision for future events as they may affect the General Hospital.

Hospitality

Spirituality

Vision

Justice

Sacredness of Life

A Town at an Impasse

In the closing years of the 19th century, as Sault Ste. Marie was transformed from a provincial town into a thriving industrial centre, it became a town in need of a modern hospital. Francis Clergue, W.H. Plummer and the town's other promoters knew that a hospital was necessary as a community centrepiece to entice investment, and as a social institution to preserve a stable workforce. How was the town to care for its citizens?

Dr. Robert Gibson and his scientifically trained peers knew the value of a professionally administered hospital, a trained staff of nurses, and a sterile operating room. In the post-Lister and post-Nightingale era, a hospital was a necessary element of good medical care. A kitchen table and a set of surgical instruments were no longer good enough.

Maria Plummer and a growing number of her urban, middle-class counterparts also believed that a hospital was necessary to care for the less fortunate among them who were devastated by sickness. Those with family support systems were well cared for — it was the increasing numbers of workers, often single men, who were flocking to the community who were left vulnerable in times of sickness.

Provisions for the indigent sick were scanty in the Sault Ste. Marie of the 1890s. The only public institution was an isolation hospital described in an 1893 issue of the *Algoma Missionary News* as

> a log shanty standing halfway between the Sault and Slabtown. It sags down a good deal on one side and you instinctively wonder how much longer it will maintain that graceful angle and how soon it will be parallel with mother earth. There is a strong iron bar across the door for it has been used as a lockup [from the old HBC post?]. There is one room 20' x 14' and in it are six beds, a stove and two tables. The place is so small that one of the patients nearly has his head in the stove; but the latter cannot be dispensed with and there is no other place for the former.[14]

With overcrowded conditions, a constant flow of travellers through town, and a poor water supply, typhoid was always a lurking problem. In 1896, after the town had incurred an expense of $1,600 to care for indigents, the time seemed right for town council to push for a modern hospital.

A committee was created, consisting of the mayor

Edward Biggings, businessman Simon John Dawson, lawyer J.J. Kehoe, George A. Hunter, and Robert Rush. Dr. Robert J. Gibson, the Sault's most prominent and forward-looking physician, provided the business acumen for the committee. This group had a formidable job ahead of them. Early in their deliberations, they were told in no uncertain terms that the extent of the town's support would be to provide a site but nothing else. When J.J. Kehoe, secretary of the committee, wrote to council to inquire of their intentions, the clerk was instructed to write back to him, thanking Kehoe for his interest but informing him, "that this Council is in favour of the town granting a site for the hospital, *but nothing more.*[15]"

Both levels of government were approached, without success. Sir Oliver Mowat's provincial Liberals were a government of minimalism, with a loathing of debt. They felt little responsibility toward the sick of the province beyond paying for the institutional care of indigents through the Charity Aid Act. There was no interest in setting a precedent and financing the building of a charitable institution in a far-off town.

The federal government could have been receptive. It had established marine hospitals in the port cities of Port Arthur, Collingwood, Owen Sound, and St. Catharines. Dr. Gibson, Mayor Biggings, and S.J. Dawson travelled to Ottawa to present their case but returned empty-handed. Sir Wilfrid Laurier's interest in Sault Ste. Marie did not include funding a hospital, and it may have been that the era of federal funding for marine hospitals was over.

The large companies and industries of the town were approached for assistance but, with the exception of Francis Clergue, they all declined. However, it is difficult to imagine who else there would have been besides Clergue to provide such assistance. Apart from government agencies and the typical entrepreneurs such as merchants, lawyers, contractors, etc., there were no wealthy industrialists in the Sault — no railway magnates, no logging or fishing enterprises, no mining millionaires. It would take another generation for the Plummer family to be in a position to donate its home, Lynnhurst, to become the Plummer Memorial Public Hospital, and for a summer visitor to St. Joseph Island, Mrs. M. Matthews, to donate the property and funds to establish Matthews Memorial Hospital.

Every possible window seemed to be closed and on the evening of May 21, 1897, the town council made a decision that left the hospital committee with only one option. That evening, the councillors met for their regular session. On the agenda was a proposal made two days previously by councillor W.H. Plummer and seconded by Councillor Sims: that council consider purchasing the newly vacated Wawanosh Home for use as a hospital. Like all city or town councils, this group took its work seriously, but they could have no idea how their decision would reverberate for the next several generations. And so, just after considering a petition to build a sidewalk along Queen Street west of Spring, council considered the Plummer proposal.

The Wawanosh Home had been a residential school for Native girls, built in 1879 on the present Great Northern Road, at the corner of Wawanosh Avenue. It was closed in 1897 when the girls were transferred to the Shingwauk Home on Queen Street (today's Algoma University College).

Had the council felt able to finance the purchase, it would have been a simple matter to turn the Home into a hospital by purchasing some beds, linen, kitchen equipment, etc., and hiring a matron and some nurses. Many hospitals across Ontario started this way, as something akin to very clean and expertly run boarding houses. Twenty years later, the Plummer

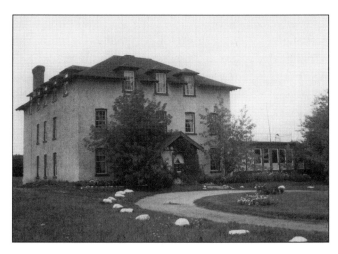

The building that almost became Sault Ste. Marie's first hospital. The Wawanosh House (later the Children's Aid Society) was at the top of Pim Street hill.
Courtesy The Sault Star

Hospital started life in a house on Albert Street before moving to the Plummer family home.

But in 1897, the Sault was on shaky financial footing, and so council turned down the Wawanosh proposal. The Home was eventually purchased in 1912 by the Children's Aid Society, which operated it as a children's shelter until 1955. Had council accepted Plummer's proposal, today there would most likely be a public hospital on Great Northern Road where the Canadian Legion building stands today.

And so with no civic support, no offers of help from the provincial or federal governments, no wealthy philanthropist, the hospital committee was at an impasse.

Interestingly, there is some evidence that while the town fathers were trying to establish a hospital, there was a parallel attempt by the town "mothers" that ended in failure. Some newspaper items suggest that a group of prominent women, including Maria Plummer and Mrs. W. Ewing, attempted to establish a hospital sponsored by the Victorian Order of Nurses.

The VON was created in 1897 as a special project of Queen Victoria's jubilee year. It was under the patronage of Lady Ishbel Aberdeen, the wife of the governor general, and VON branches were being created across the country, generally administered by volunteer boards of interested women.

The *Sault Express* reported that one summer Sunday, in 1897, Lord and Lady Aberdeen arrived unannounced at St. Andrew's Presbyterian (now United) Church for the evening service. They were recognized by several members of the congregation and welcomed by the minister, William A. Duncan. (Duncan was the father of Sault physician Dr. John H. Duncan). The Aberdeens seem to have come to town at the request of Dr. Gibson to discuss a proposal with Gibson, Mrs. Ewing, and Mrs. Plummer to establish a VON hospital. Nothing came of the Sault leg of the visit; however, their trip had at least one success: a VON hospital was established later that year in Thessalon, just east of the Sault.

Portrait

Dr. Robert James Gibson

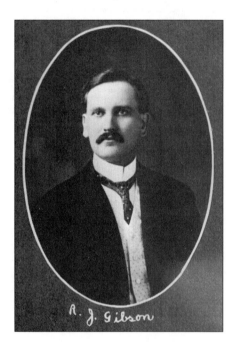

Dr. Robert Gibson, "the father of the General Hospital."

Today he is all but forgotten, but in the early years of the century, Dr. Robert James Gibson was justly known as the "father of the General Hospital." He was a remarkable man, skilled as a physician, energetic in his promotion of the hospital, and interested always in the good of the wider community.

Gibson was born near Guelph on the eve of Confederation on November 10, 1866. He was educated in Clinton in the new province of Ontario, and he graduated with his MD from McGill University in 1892. Following graduation, Gibson did what only the elite medical students of his day could do — he travelled to Great Britain for postgraduate work at the University of Edinburgh, home of Joseph Lister.

On his return to Canada in 1893, Gibson was engaged for about a year by the Canadian Pacific Railway as a company physician stationed in Chapleau. In 1894, the same year Francis Clergue arrived, Gibson set up practice in Sault Ste. Marie. He may have been influenced by the Clergue hoopla; he was probably also influenced by his future brother-in-law Dr. J. Reid, who was a CPR physician based in the Sault. To an energetic and ambitious young man like Gibson, the Sault must have seemed a natural place to establish a surgical practice.

At the age of 31, in 1897, Gibson married Jenny Marks of Bruce Mines, which was at this time declining from its heyday as Canada's richest copper town. It had boasted a population of 1,500 in the 1860s and had taken some $7,000,000 in copper from its three mines. Jenny Marks and her sister Annie (Marks) Reid were daughters of one of the Marks brothers, Bruce Mines' major merchants, and cousins of Maria (Wiley) Plummer. Gibson was thus related by marriage to the Sault's most esteemed doctor, J. Reid, and most powerful merchant, W.H. Plummer.

Together, James and Jenny built a beautiful residence at the northwest corner of Brock and Albert Streets, directly across from St. Luke's Cathedral. Until the house was built, his office was located in a house on East Street. He is credited with having the first x-ray machine in northern Ontario "run by water power" installed in his office.

On arrival in Sault Ste. Marie, Gibson entered wholeheartedly into the struggle to establish a hospital. His letters to the Grey Sisters in Ottawa show a complete grasp of what was necessary to bring the hospital to reality, and he even felt comfortable writing to Ottawa to comment on his preference for the next mother superior at the hospital.

Always interested in the advancement of his profession, Gibson served for twelve years on the executive of the Ontario Medical Council, was part of a small group of physicians who prepared the legislation to form the Dominion Medical Council, and served on that council's executive. He ran unsuccessfully as the Liberal candidate in the 1910 federal election but served on the Sault's High School Board for many years, chairing it at the time of his unexpected death in 1919

During the Great War of 1914 –1918, Gibson served as captain in the Canadian Army Medical Corps. Demobilized in December of 1918, he returned to his Sault practice but died eight months later of a heart attack, three months from his 54th birthday. He was predeceased by one son but was survived by his wife Jenny, and another son, Robert.

Gibson also left behind a community greatly enriched by his work. The *Sault Star* commented that he was "actively identified with the public and social life of the city, more particularly with the General Hospital where he was the head surgeon and where he was recognized as a most generous physician."[16] One of his peers eulogised him by saying, "Seldom in the history of the place has the death of one of its citizens caused such deep regret as the death of Dr. Gibson. He has, however, left to the citizens of this City the precious memory of a great and good man, a beautiful character and a life devoted to service."[17] In tribute after his death, the new General Hospital nurses' wing, completed in 1923, was named in his honour.

Grey Sisters Answer the Call

Grey Sisters Answer the Call

All of the usual avenues had been exhausted. The delegation who travelled to Ottawa to request funding for a marine hospital had been turned down. The provincial government saw its role only as paying a stipend for indigent care, certainly not as funding the construction of hospitals across the province. The town council had been wary of committing itself for the ownership and maintenance of a hospital building. The Sault's finances were precarious enough without taking on the running of an institution. The hospital committee was at a standstill.

Finally, on June 28, 1897, a breakthrough occurred. T.F. Chamberlain, the provincial inspector of asylums and prisons, visiting the Sault on one of his regular inspection tours, met with the hospital committee. "If you wish a hospital of which the work is serious and lasting," he is reported to have said to the committee, "ask the Grey Sisters."

Provincial government archives are silent as to who Chamberlain was and how he knew of the work of the Grey Sisters, but two possibilities are likely. He may have come from Ottawa and knew of the work of the sisters at Ottawa General. But more likely, since Sudbury would also have been on his inspection circuit, he would have first-hand knowledge of their

work. There, in 1896, they had taken an old two-storey CPR hospital and turned it into a clean, modern hospital to serve the nickel miners who were surging into town.

If little is known about Chamberlain himself, a description of his job gives a good snapshot of emerging views of health care. Eight years before Confederation, in 1859, the united provinces of Canada East and West took a tiny first step toward administering public institutions by creating the Board of Inspectors of Asylums and Prisons. At the time, there were sixty-one public institutions: fifty-two common jails, four lunatic asylums, three penitentiaries, and only two hospitals.

At the time of Confederation, this board was reaffirmed with the Prisons and Asylums Inspection Act. The inspector's responsibility was for the "peace, welfare and good government" of these institutions and this was accomplished by framing by-laws and making twice-yearly inspection visits to examine the books and operations. The inspectors' yearly reports trace a growing awareness that hospitals and asylums were different from prisons and reformatories, which in turn were different from orphanages and rest homes. By 1893 there were three inspectors, of whom Chamberlain was one.

Hospital administration became an increasingly important part of the Board's workload and there were a number of administrative shifts. Finally, in 1930, hospitals were transferred to the Department of Health (with the Sault's H.M. Robbins as the first deputy minister).

Chamberlain's recommendation was all the encouragement the committee needed and they entered negotiations immediately with the Grey Sisters. The following day, June 29, 1897, Dr. Gibson wrote to Sister St. Cyprien, a Grey Sister working at St. Joseph's Hospital in Sudbury. St. Cyprien had already visited the town, probably on a hospital "begging tour" to the surrounding lumber camps. Gibson's letter demonstrates his grasp of what was needed to establish a hospital: a site, furnishings, and an assured source of operating funds. He leaves out the cost of the building, which he expects the religious order to assume.

> A visit from Dr. Chamberlain last night revived the idea of having or attempting to have your order establish a hospital at this place. He thinks that this would be a much better place to build than in Sudbury, provided the town would give substantial financial and moral support, which I am satisfied it would do in the first place. They [the council] have already voted a site, benevolent societies and others have promised to furnish about 20 beds and I believe the town would give an annual grant of say $300 toward maintenance, then a large revenue could be derived from the camps about here and from neighboring municipalities, then of course there would be the usual government grant. I would like very much if you could visit the town again, I

> would have a meeting of the council called and would call a meeting of hospital committee and thus come to some definite arrangement. Of course I am very anxious to see a hospital established and from what I know of hospitals managed by the community to which you belong, I have no doubt but that you would be very strongly supported by all classes of the district. Dr. Chamberlain is writing to your Superior General at Ottawa. You will probably do so too. As you are acquainted with our circumstances, what is wanted is a building, the rest will easily by supplied.
>
> Thanking you for the very kind interest you have taken in this project already and hoping for a continuance of your good wishes.[18]

Mail travelled quickly in those days! The very next day, June 30, 1897, Sr. St. Raphael (most likely the mother superior in Sudbury) wrote to Superior General Demers in Ottawa, enclosing the previous day's letter from Dr. Gibson with her own and mentioning that Chamberlain would be sending his recommendation in writing to her in Ottawa. She begins by noting that the people of Sault Ste. Marie "have not abandoned the project of having a hospital under the control of the Grey Sisters of Ottawa." (This statement is similar to the reference by Gibson to the discussion he and Sr. St. Cyprien had already had about such a move.) "You will remember, my dear Mother," she continues, "having written to me that you would accept a hospital perhaps in the Sault, perhaps in North Bay, after which my Sr. St. Cyprien has met with Dr. Gibson and given him the understanding that if he addresses [the matter] to our Congregation, he would be able to have the Sisters to direct their hospital; it is with this hope that he has begun the project." She closes the letter by saying that she and Sr. St. Cyprien, "await your <u>decisive</u> response."[19]

The letter is of interest for another piece of information that she passes on: "Here" she writes, "people tell us that the Sault is a place of the future." J.A. Primeau, Jesuit priest at Sacred Heart (now Precious Blood Cathedral), also wrote encouragingly to Superior General Demers, saying that he was very much in favour of the sisters taking on the hospital project and assuring her that, "the citizens, in great majority Protestant, are strongly in favour of a hospital established by the Sisters and are disposed to assist."[20] He suggested that the two could meet later in the summer when he was returning from a pilgrimage to Ste. Anne de Beaupré. Fr. Primeau concludes by suggesting that the sisters may also wish to be involved in education in the Sault. The Grey Sisters did not take up this challenge, although they must have considered it. (There is an interesting exchange of letters between the Sisters and the Francis Clergue estate over the purchase of his home for the establishment of a college.)

Over the next year, the Grey Sisters must indeed have made a decisive response, so that in May of 1898, Dr. Gibson was able to report to the new superior general, Sr. Dorothy Kirby, that he had just presented to council "your proposal to build a hospital here and asked for their assistance. They unanimously agreed to furnish a site and they appointed a committee to select and purchase the same, provided you could be induced to locate here."

He continued with a discussion of sites. Gibson's preference was "a beautiful location on the hill [which] has sewer and water pipes past it" and which was known as the "old high school site." The preference of Fr. Primeau was a waterfront location just down the street from the church. "Its only advantage is that it is a little easier of access than the other on account of there being no hill to climb." Fr. Primeau's waterfront preference carried the day. It was most likely the more popular location since most hospitals of the day were being constructed near water or in open, airy locations because of the beneficial effects of the air. However the "hospital on the hill" concept has remained popular among Saultites. As recently as the 1960s, there was a proposal to scrap both hospitals and build from scratch on the hill.

Gibson also refers in the letter to "the crippled state of the town's finances" and says, "I took it upon myself to say to the Council that if they could not afford to purchase the site outright at present that you would assume the debt, they to pay $100 annually until the whole was paid." In other words, town finances in 1898 were in such perilous shape that the council was asking the sisters to hold the mortgage on the lot as well as the building.

He comments on an architectural drawing, which has already been sent to Fr. Primeau, and tells the superior general that although he likes it very much he feels that a smaller building would suffice and "if built on the wing plan, it could be added to when necessary." Dr. Gibson did not know how accurately he was predicting the future, nor could he know that twenty-four years later a new east wing nurses' residence would be named and dedicated to his memory. He closes the letter by assuring Sr. Kirby that, "any service I can do you will be done cheerfully."[21]

Several days later, on June 3, 1898, Superior General Kirby writes to Fr. Primeau that her board has decided to undertake the work, "even at the price of sacrifices that it will be necessary to make." She expresses the desire that if the building cannot be completed quickly, they would like to rent a house and begin their hospital work immediately.

Negotiations began immediately over the design of the hospital and the purchase of the site, and a flurry of letters passed back and forth between Fr. Primeau and Mother Kirby. J.J. Kehoe, one of the members of the hospital committee, recommended that it would be prudent to purchase the riverfront lot immediately. He was afraid that the owners would raise their asking price, hoping that the Grand Trunk Railway would be constructing a new rail line in the area (two of that company's directors had just been to visit the town). Finally, negotiations were completed and three lots were purchased, one for $1,000, the other two for $850 and $875, all with rights to the water lot. Fr. Primeau congratulated Mère Kirby on an excellent purchase and Kehoe wrote to her, "I may say that I think the property is the most desirable that you could have in town and you cannot fail to be pleased with its location."

Architect James Thomson (offices in the Vaughan Block on Queen Street) sent architectural drawings to Ottawa, pointing out "several features which I consider commendable in a hospital building, viz. every part of the building, especially the wards gets free circulation of air on three sides, the administrative part convenient to and yet sufficiently removed from the wards, the kitchen and private rooms also well removed, good bathroom accommodation, the building so arranged that it could be easily enlarged by the addition of another wing."[22]

These matters settled, attention turned to fundraising in the lumbercamps. and Dr. Gibson suggested quick action in a letter to Mère Kirby:

> The Niagara Falls Pulp & Paper Co. are putting in five camps near here next week. May I suggest having tickets ready as soon as possible so that agents for other hospitals will not get the field ahead of you.

Mr. Thomas Bishop (manager for above Company) spoke to me some time ago re the selling of tickets, he said he would handle them himself for a commission the amount was not mentioned, he would be a good man as he has the employment and paying of all the men. Other camps will be opening up very soon, so that someone should be on the spot.[23]

Fr. Primeau also wrote to say that, "a Mr. Sullivan, a good Catholic, asked to have charge of selling the tickets in the lumber camps."[24]

The House on Water Street

The House on Water Street

Finally the big day had arrived. On September 13, 1898, the two sisters chosen as foundresses for the new hospital arrived in Sault Ste. Marie on the 6:30 evening train. The speed and ease of their journey stood in stark contrast to that of four Grey Sisters some fifty years earlier who had rested at Sault Ste. Marie on their way from Montreal to the Red River settlement. That journey had been by freighter canoe with a Hudson's Bay party and several priests. The journey had taken fifty-nine days and the nuns' luggage had travelled via England to Hudson Bay, then overland to St. Boniface.

Sr. Marie du Sauveur and Sr. Ste. Rosalie, the hospital's foundresses, travelled from Ottawa to Sault Ste. Marie by train, probably stopping off to visit their sisters at St. Joseph's Hospital in Sudbury. They were met at the station by Mrs. O'Brien, a former pupil from Pembroke, who offered them the hospitality of the family's home for several days until they took possession of the house that would serve as a temporary hospital.

On their first visit to the construction site, the sisters remarked on a fact that has continued to plague the General Hospital through the years — the high water-table in a site so close to the river.

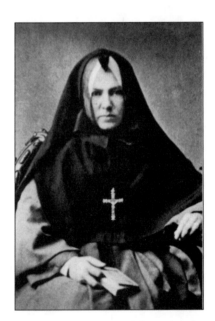

Marie du Sauveur, foundress and first administrator of the General Hospital.   **Courtesy SCO**

Construction was not proceeding as quickly as hoped because, in many areas, the land was quicksand. In places, the construction company was digging twelve feet for foundations.

There is no record of a precise address on Water (now Bay) Street where the sisters set up their first hospital. However, it must have been in the vicinity of the government dock, to the west of Ermatinger's stone home. Edward Capp's 1904 book, *The Story of Bawating: Being the Annals of Sault Ste. Marie* calls it, "a modest house on Bay Street near Pim." Various documents state that it was brick, that it was previously occupied by three families, and that by the 1930s it had been torn down. Fr. Primeau had negotiated the rental ($15 per month) on the sisters' behalf.

Whatever the exact location, the sisters found the house to be very unsatisfactory for a hospital, the lower floor being "damp and unhealthy." However, having no choice, they moved in and resolutely set about to arrange it as efficiently as possible. At the end of September, Marie du Sauveur and Ste. Rosalie were joined by Sr. Ste. Désiré and Sr. St. Pacifique, the latter becoming the cook. Through the first year, they cared for usually seven or eight patients at a time (a total of twenty-two by Christmas). Four physicians — Drs. Gibson, McCaig, Reid, and Flemming — took turns (week about) in providing medical care. Men were cared for on the first floor, women on the second. The operating table was on the first floor, and a Native student from Shingwauk School was the first patient to have surgery (his left leg was amputated by Dr. Gibson).

Typhoid was a terrifying presence in the town in those years. The sisters' *Chroniques* report that the first patient was a typhoid victim who was received on September 23. The patient, Alice Reynolds, was a young woman of 22, part of a travelling theatre troupe. Dr. Flemming cared for her and a second typhoid victim, Joseph Therien, admitted two days later. They were unable to find anyone willing to come in and do the laundry for fear of contracting typhoid, and so the sisters did the laundry themselves at night and hung the sheets to dry around the stove.

The sisters spent ten months, until July 1899, coping with these difficult arrangements. Through the winter there was frost on the walls. There was very little space for the sisters to live, and the two younger nuns slept in the garrett. There was no water connection in the house and they transported water by barrels from the river's edge. The hospital's beds arrived by boat sometime during the summer. The *Chroniques* note that, during their stay in the temporary hospital, sixty-four patients were cared for and there were three deaths.

Moving to Queen Street

Moving to Queen Street

The cornerstone of the new hospital building was laid on Wednesday, September 21, 1898. It was a momentous event for the young town, "un grand fla fla," as one of the Grey Sisters remarked. In his comments, Mayor Edward Biggings noted that this was the opening of the town's first public charitable institution.

Many of the Sault's prominent citizens were in attendance — along with Mayor Biggings, there was the entire town council: W.H. Plummer, who had headed up town council's Hospital Committee, W.G. Sims, Edmund Parr, I. Taillefer, R.M. Van Norman, William Graham, and Robert Lang. Contractors W.J. Thompson and John O'Boyle were in attendance, as was C.F. Farwell, KC, provincial member of parliament for Algoma. Among the clergy were Father Primeau, from Sacred Heart parish, who had acted as the agent of the Grey Sisters in the Sault, Fathers Macdonald and Côté, both Jesuits, and also the Presbyterian and Baptist ministers.

The ceremonies were conducted by the man who had done the most to make the hospital a reality — Dr. Robert J. Gibson. In his speech, Gibson reviewed the struggle made by the townspeople to secure a hospital and the answer to the call by the Grey Sisters. He stressed that although "the institution would be under the management of the Sisters, its doors would be open to the black and the white, the rich and poor, the Protestant and Catholic alike ...The afternoon's proceedings were of such a cordial character" concludes the newspaper account, "as to cement more closely together than they have ever been before the Roman Catholics and Protestants of the Soo in the bonds of social relationship and sympathetic friendship."[25] An offering of $40 was collected in support of the hospital.

The building was ready for occupancy by July 1899, and the original four sisters were quickly joined by five of their comrades from Ottawa — Marie de l'Annunciation, Leopold, St. Fortunat, Heliodore, and Apolline.

The grand opening of the hospital was a joyous affair held on September 28, 1899, almost exactly one year after the nuns' arrival. Superior General Kirby attended from Ottawa, and Sr. St. Raphael, mother superior at St. Joseph's Hospital in Sudbury, also came. The day began with mass in the hospital's chapel, presided over by Father Primeau with the assistance of Fathers McDonald, Chambon, Côté and Lamarche. At night, there was a reception organized by the Ladies' Auxiliary, and from 7:00 onwards, the

Chroniques report, "the house [hospital] was lit up from top to bottom, all the doors were open and a great crowd visited the nooks and crannies of the house and each one pronounced themselves enchanted with the visit."[26]

An early newspaper, *The Reporter*, edited by H.R. Halton, gave a detailed description of this earliest hospital building. Note the combination of traditional hospital features — public wards, bedrooms for live-in help — and modern innovations — private rooms for paying patients, a pathology lab, x-ray machine. (Halton's description contrasts somewhat with the hospital reminiscences of Sr. Ste. Constance, reprinted elsewhere.)

There are ten strictly private rooms, elegantly furnished and the rooms in which from two to four patients are placed, as well as the public wards, are scrupulously clean.

The kitchen, pantries and bath rooms are equipped with every convenience and device known to sanitary science. The operating room is a model of its kind, with every appliance necessary in surgery. The rooms are so arranged that fever patients, surgery cases and those suffering from chronic diseases are entirely separate, and contagious diseases can be perfectly isolated, and rigid quarantine maintained.

Not the least inviting part of the hospital is the pretty little chapel, in which mass is said every day except Sunday and which is always open to the patients who are able to go there to pray.

The basement contains the kitchen, sisters' dining room, small dining room for help, furnace room, helps' bedrooms and storage room. The first floor includes ten large and well-furnished private wards, a dispensary, general waiting room, physician's waiting room, and large recreation room for the sisters. Off this floor are three large verandahs, which are of great benefit to convalescent patients in helping to restore them to renewed health and vigor.

The second floor consists of two private rooms, a small ward of eight beds for women and a large public ward, which, however, is so well ventilated and lighted that when necessary the number of beds can be increased without any inconvenience. Off the large ward is a small room which is used as a rule for very sick patients from the public ward, their removal from which during this period being a matter of no small comfort not only to the patient himself but also to his fellow sufferers. On this floor also is a small but very complete little laboratory for the physicians' use, where they can pursue their researches in urinalysis, microscopic work, etc., a convenience of inestimable value aiding the physician to be more thorough in his work and to keep abreast with the times in the diagnosing and treatment of his cases.... Near to the laboratory we have a room given entirely to a late addition to our very thorough equipment, namely the x-ray department, which as has been said has become a necessity in every large general hospital. This consists of a large fourteen plate machine with a full line of appliances in connection for the production of the Rontgen rays and the generating of static electricity, which is used so frequently now in the treatment of many forms of nervous diseases and paralysis.... On this floor also is a small but beautiful little chapel which is a great convenience to the sisters and many of the patients. There are also in connection with this floor two open verandahs, where convalescent patients can receive the benefit of sun and fresh air.

The third floor consists of a public surgical ward of eight beds with five private wards, which, however are used for either female surgical cases or serious operative cases which require special attention. There is also a well equipped dressing room or emergency operating room and a thoroughly lighted and well appointed operating room for major operations, which is a credit to the hospital and gives facilities to the surgeons for doing aseptic work such as are not to be found outside of a hospital and which is a most essential factor in all surgical work.... The sisters' dormitory is also on this floor and is large and well ventilated as are also all rooms and wards in the buildings. The halls and stairs are all laid with rubber matting, the work of the Ladies' Auxiliary.[27]

To have successfully opened a hospital by 1898 places Sault Ste. Marie in the ranks of the established cities and towns of Ontario. The 1898 Report of the Inspector of Prisons and Public Charities upon the Hospitals of the Province of Ontario states that there were forty-eight hospitals in operation across the province and that "hospitals are now pretty fairly established in all the cities and towns of the Province." The small number of hospitals across the north attests to the area's sparse population: there were hospitals only in Ottawa, Pembroke, Mattawa, Sudbury, Port Arthur, and Rat Portage (Kenora). All were Catholic, three belonging to the Grey Sisters and two to the Sisters of St. Joseph. All except Sudbury were towns that owed their beginnings to the fur trade.

Inspector T.F. Chamberlain, the inspector of prisons and public charities, who had been so influential in bringing the Grey Sisters to the Sault, paid his first visit to the General Hospital in August 1900. He complimented the sisters on their hospital and expressed his view that every hospital run by the Grey Sisters seemed always to be in excellent condition.

New Wings for a Growing Community

New Wings for a Growing Community

No sooner was the hospital opened than it seemed to be too small, and agitation began to construct a new wing. The Sault was booming. In the ten years from 1893 to 1903, the population quadrupled — from 2,000 to 8,000. Almost half were Clergue workers.

The great infectious diseases of the 19th century were always a threat, and as the town industrialized it became more vulnerable to epidemics. Workers for the new Clergue industries swelled the town. Travellers passing through, sailors from the Great Lakes freighters, and shantymen from the many nearby lumber camps could easily bring typhoid, smallpox, or diphtheria into town. The staff, doctors, and facilities at the General Hospital were being taxed to the limit.

A 1902 *Sault Star* article titled "Hospital Wing Badly Needed" described the situation. Dr. Gimby had brought the problem to town council, warning them that the hospital's halls and reception areas were "full of beds and it was impossible to get a patient into the institution."[28]

Fr. T. Lussier, the new Jesuit priest at Sacred Heart Church, echoed the same sentiments in a letter to the superior general in Ottawa, telling her that the hospital was crowded with the sick "even in the parlour" and the sisters were unable to give the care they would like to give. This potential for instability in the workforce was of concern to company investors, and Lussier's purpose in writing Superior General Kirby was to tell her that Francis Clergue had offered to donate $5,000 and enough sandstone to build an addition to the hospital — preferably in front of the current building since Clergue considered the hospital's red-brick exterior "disappointing." In the same letter, Lussier reported that Clergue had also spoken to him of an American company that had offered to build and equip a new Sault hospital at a cost of $100,000 if they could be assured of having an exclusive arrangement to treat all Clergue employees. Clergue had told them that he was not interested — the Grey Sisters had arrived first and their work was most satisfactory; he would not support a hospital in opposition.

Lussier urged the sisters to consider building the addition. "L'avenir du Sault, je crois, est assure" — the future of the Sault is solid, he wrote, and went on to describe the Jesuits' own plans to build a school and a college.

At the same time, there was renewed interest in

building a non-denominational hospital. Sectarian feeling was never far from the surface in 19th century Ontario, and the argument was put forward that government funding would be more easily available for such a hospital. A 1907 *Sault Star* article reports that a group of benevolent societies were planning to purchase a lot at the top of the North Street hill to erect a new hospital (again, the 'hospital on the hill' plan). The argument did have its lighter moments. During one council meeting, Alderman Dawson suggested that the hospital should report each patient to his or her minister. No, replied Dr. Gimby, ministers as a rule stayed too long with their parishioners, and physicians would have more success in curing hospital cases if more quietness could be secured. He was not being disrespectful, Dr. Gimby stressed, he was only speaking as experience had taught him.

Finally in 1908, the long-anticipated west wing was completed. The addition was red brick, similar in style to the original building but with a few more gracious touches. The architect was Henry Westlake Angus, partner to James Thomson. A Canadian architectural *Who's Who* lists hospitals in Sudbury and North Bay as also being among Angus's designs. O'Boyle Bros. was the contractor, and the cost of the addition was in the range of $60,000. This addition, known as the medical wing, effectively doubled the size of the hospital. For the first time there was a children's ward, located on the fourth floor, "a pretty, cheerful room having a splendid view of the river eastward to Topsail Island,"[29] which opened onto one of the sun porches. The Ladies' Auxiliary paid for the installation of a telephone system. Plans were to conduct most patient care in the new building and to use the old wing to house, among other things, a school of nursing, or as the *Sault Star* account of the opening put it, to provide "pleasant quarters for the training school for

nurses that the sisters intend opening next autumn. This will be a great boon to young ladies of the district intending to take up the nursing profession, as the Grey Nuns are considered among the best nurses to be had anywhere and hitherto those girls desiring this training had to go to distant cities to acquire it."[30]

The medical wing was inaugurated with a gala opening ceremony on June 15, 1908. Again, Dr. Gibson, "the father of the hospital," officiated at the ceremonies in which, said the *Sault Star*, "the beautiful grounds were gaily decorated and a blazing semicircle of electric lights looked like a scene from fairyland."

In 1912, the year Sault Ste. Marie incorporated as a city and the Algoma Steel Corp. was formed, the General Hospital quietly and perhaps unknowingly became a modern hospital — that is, it became a core community institution, an essential part of a modern industrial city. The hospital's financial position had always been perilous and was becoming more so as surgery became more sophisticated, and expensive equipment had to be upgraded. In that year, the new president of Algoma Steel, J. Frater Taylor, proposed forming a group of gentlemen who would "look after the financial interest of the hospital." The superior general concurred, and Taylor took on the chairmanship of this board, which called itself the Special Finance Committee. Thus, the beginnings of what would become the modern hospital advisory board.

The committee included Taylor and A.H. Chitty from Algoma Steel; Drs. Gibson, McLean, and McQuaid, MPP; C.N. Smith; Mayor Wm. H. Munro; H.E. Talbott, president of the Lake Superior Paper Co. (who was at that time living in the Clergue mansion Montfermier); W.E. Franz from the Algoma Central Railway; J.A. Hussey from Spanish River Pulp & Paper; and J. Lyons. They published a little booklet, *Let us Lift the Burden from the Sault Ste. Marie General Hospital*, which contained a detailed hospital balance sheet. The booklet was distributed to all Sault businesses with a letter urging workers and owners to donate to the hospital. The *Chroniques* note that the campaign brought in $8,000, enough to pay the hospital's outstanding debts with the exception of the $40,000 mortgage.

Sault Ste. Marie had become a stable community with a reasonably diverse economy. By 1918 the population had reached 21,500. A sizeable middle class brought with it one of that group's best features, a social conscience, a belief that it was possible, through diligence and hard work, to make life better for everyone in the community. The opening of the Royal Victoria (soon to be Plummer) Hospital in 1917 was an expression of this community-mindedness. The work of the Women's Institutes in establishing the Thessalon and Matthews Memorial Hospitals in the early 1920s were expressions of a social conscience as well. The General Hospital Ladies Auxiliary's 1914 project — to raise funds for improvements to the kitchen — was typical of a stalwart middle class pulling together to improve life.

The *Algoma Pioneer* reported the June 1914 meeting as, "a good meeting, all prepared to do their duty.... The proposed garden party in aid of the building fund for the hospital kitchen ... will be one of the largest and best planned ever held on the lovely lawns of the hospital if the present ideal weather prevails. An excellent and varied programme in which some of the best known singers and musicians of the Soo will take part will be given on the great western porch which will be artistically decorated and lighted up for the occasion.... And so it goes all along the line, improvement everywhere." The rationale for all of this effort? "As saving life is considered the greatest economic gain of the day, citizens will be glad and ready to help the auxiliary in their brave attempt to fight off the King of Terrors by all that modern science can do for disease in an up-to-date modern hospital kitchen under the care of a skilled and willing management."[31]

Through the war years and on into the 1920s, the General Hospital quietly soldiered on, out of the news except for the lengthy listing each year of the donations to the patients' Christmas dinner and reports of the fundraising special events held by the Ladies' Auxiliary. Most reports state that about twelve sisters managed the hospital, generally caring for forty patients. They employed lay people as laundry, kitchen and maintenance workers. There were generally two nuns who were nurses and two sisters who supervised the approximately ten student nurses. The other sisters held positions such as bookkeeper, kitchen supervisor, laundry supervisor, and pharmacist.

A typical patient of the day would have been Mr. Thurlow MacCallum from Paltimore, Quebec, who in September 1923 was brought by boat from Pukaskwa with an axe injury to his foot. Mr. MacCallum had hired on with the Lake Superior Pulp & Paper Co. to earn money to enter dentistry at McGill University. He was brought to the General on September 20, registered as patient #1014, treated by Dr. S. Casselman, and discharged on September 29. His bill (amount not noted) was paid by Workman's Compensation. Many years later, in 1983, Mr. MacCallum spent his final days at the General. At the time, his daughter, Morna Rupert, held the position of risk management coordinator, one of many hospital positions undreamed of in the 1920s.

A small (twenty-by-twenty-five-foot) washroom wing was added to the south side of the hospital in 1921, at a cost of $7,500. Renovations to the main building at the same time added a doctors' scrub room adjacent to the operating room ("perfectly immaculate, all sterilized and pure white"), redecorated the nursery, and enlarged the doctors' boardroom. Added to the boardroom were photographs of Sault doctors who had died, including Drs. J.H. Gimby, Reid, McQuaid, and Gibson.

Dr. Gibson's death in 1919 was a great blow to the community. His leadership had been crucial in bringing the General Hospital into existence and immediately there was a great community desire to honour his memory. The epidemic of Spanish flu had just ended and there was a fear that the town did not have enough trained nurses to see it through a similar crisis. Professional nurses had proved themselves invaluable during the war years and through the flu epidemic. What better way to honour Dr. Gibson's memory than with a "nurses' home" bearing his name, to be built on the hospital property?

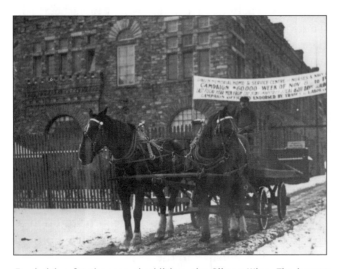

Fundraising for the second addition, the Gibson Wing. The banner reads in part, "Gibson Memorial Home & Service Centre ... Campaign $60,000 ... Campaign officially endorsed by Trades & Labor Council." The photo is taken in front of the present St. Marys Paper building. **Courtesy SSM Museum**

Funding for the home would come completely from the community. The fundraising campaign was added on to the Algoma War Chest, a fundraising effort begun during the war years. It was conducted like a military campaign under the direction of Col. C.H.L. Jones, general manager of the Spanish River Pulp & Paper Co. The "Gibson Memorial Home and Service Centre for Nurses" was to be owned by the community through a board of trustees but controlled and managed by the hospital administrator. Col. Jones told his audiences that they were "face to face with a present threat against the community's health and vital well-being ... [as] there are not enough registered nurses to properly serve the community's needs in this direction in or outside of its hospitals."[32]

The community gave generously, and the wing was commissioned in 1923. The architect was Findlay & Foulis, the contractor was J.J. Fitzpatrick, and the cost of the project was documented at $25,630. But there was a strategic error in Col. Jones's battle plan, and the committee ended its campaign with a shortfall of $15,000. Once again, the sisters' calmness in the face of financial pressures saw the crisis through. A flurry of letters went back and forth between Jones, the sisters' council in Ottawa, and J.A. Hussey, the Gibson Home vice president. The sisters made their terms clear — they would complete and maintain the building but only after having "a written document or deed by which you will give the ownership of Gibson Memorial Nurses' Home to the Community of the Grey Nuns of the Cross."[33] The committee agreed, the Gibson Home became the Gibson Wing, the sisters took on the $15,000 debt, and the building was finally completed.

The Wing was formally opened on February 16, 1925 with Col. Jones chairing the proceedings. Speeches were made by Mayor James Dawson, J.A. Hussey from the campaign committee, and Dr. McLean, who eulogized Dr. Gibson as "the most noble of men, not only as a citizen, but as physician and surgeon. To know him was to admire him and respect him."

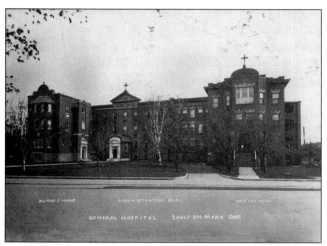

A postcard showing the old hospital with the Gibson wing completed.

The wing could accommodate about twenty nurses, with the nurses' parlour on the main floor, bedrooms and library on the second floor, and laboratory "fitted out most completely" in the basement. The physicians donated equipment, including "a magnificent microscope valued at $120." The area previously occupied by the nurses was turned into a maternity ward that "rivalled the institutions of the great cities."[34]

There was no further building of any magnitude for another thirty years, until the New Pavilion was completed in 1954. By that time, the General Hospital had new owners, and the city was coping with a more pleasant epidemic — the great 20th century epidemic of births known as the baby boom.

Portrait

The 1918 Flu Epidemic

Everyone who remembers the polio epidemic of the 1950s will understand the terror that gripped Canada in the fall of 1918 as the Spanish Flu (part of a worldwide pandemic) swept from east to west across the country. The virus was carried to North America by soldiers returning from the Great War. It attacked suddenly and its victims were mainly healthy young adults. Over the six months from September, 1918 to April, 1919, this virulent flu claimed more lives than had the Great War itself. In Sault Ste. Marie, the General Hospital and its one-year-old counterpart the Royal Victoria Hospital, had their mettle tested.

The first victim in Sault Ste. Marie was a young man working in a lumber camp around Searchmont. On October 18, 1918, the *Sault Star* reported that "two serious cases were brought down from Searchmont in a boxcar last night and were removed to the General Hospital. The men were so sick that it was impossible to let them stay at Searchmont without full medical treatment .... They were transported in an auto truck to the hospital."[35] The paper reported the death of one of the young men the next day. He was not quite 15 years old.

The crisis was ably handled by the medical officer of health, Dr. A.S. McCaig, who banned public gatherings including theatre presentations and church services, instituted rigid quarantines, and stopped ferry traffic from Sault Ste. Marie, Michigan. McCaig even gave his office over for use as an emergency headquarters, and he has been credited with guiding Sault Ste. Marie through the epidemic with common sense and wisdom.

The Sault was fortunate to have two well-run

hospitals to care for the most severe cases. Nurses were crucially needed to care for the sick, and enormous credit must go to the nuns, the other hospital nurses, and to the many women who came forward to volunteer (and many times to be quarantined with a family coping with the disease). Dr. McCaig issued a public call for nurses, both to "assist in the hospitals or assist experienced nurses in other places when the hospital accommodation has been taken up." It was agreed that ten dollars per week would be an appropriate amount if people wished to pay. The Imperial Order Daughters of the Empire (founded 1900) offered to coordinate the volunteer nursing and meals service, and the Knights of Columbus offered their meeting hall as an isolation hospital.

The *Chroniques* noted, "The terrible epidemic of so called Spanish Influenza broke out in the city and the hospital in a few days was taxed to the utmost capacity. The Good Sisters of St. Joseph and the Sisters of Wisdom, through their respective superiors, were the first to volunteer their services to aid our Sisters and nurses to cope with the disease. [The schools were ordered closed early in November.] Dr. McCaig, health officer, also procured outside nurses. High school teachers volunteered to help even in the diet kitchen."[36]

The record goes on to note three sisters who fell sick with the flu and on November 8, the *Sault Star* reported the death of Miss Florence Gibeau a helper at the General Hospital. (One of the first deaths in Canada had been of a nun at the Hôtel-Dieu in Montreal.) The epidemic seemed to peak in late November, just at the time of the armistice, when many disregarded the ban on public gatherings and took to the streets to celebrate the war's end.

In an interview on his retirement, Dr. McCaig recalled that there had been seventy-five deaths in Sault Ste. Marie from the epidemic, and he called it the worst ever to hit the city. On a personal level, the legacy of the epidemic was tragic. But it succeeded in focusing the country's attention on health as a governmental responsibility. Within months of the passing of the epidemic and the signing of the armistice, the federal Department of Health was created. "At this time" noted one parliamentarian, "when the value of human life has become of greatest moment, it is fitting that the House and the country should turn attention to considering better measures for conserving the health of our people."

In Sault Ste. Marie, the epidemic had a second impact. It made the community realize the importance of a supply of trained nurses, and it led directly to the fundraising for the Gibson Memorial Home for Nurses.

A Change of Ownership

The year of 1926 was bittersweet for the General Hospital: the hospital said a sad good-bye to its foundresses, the Grey Nuns of the Cross (Sisters of Charity) but welcomed its new owners, a newly minted religious order, the Grey Sisters of the Immaculate Conception. When the hospital was established in 1898, there was a strong French-speaking presence in Sault Ste. Marie. The French-speaking days of the fur trade were still within recent memory. Most of the sisters were francophone, the priests at Sacred Heart spoke and wrote to them in French, and all of the correspondence with the Ottawa motherhouse was in French. But as it industrialized, the town was changing into an anglophone community — the doctors had names like McCaig, Gibson, Gimby, McLean, and Fleming. Repeatedly, newspaper articles refer to Sault Ste. Marie as being a mainly Protestant town. It was natural that in the terms of the separation, the hospital would be given to the English-speaking Grey Sisters of the Immaculate Conception.

The loss of the hospital was a bitter blow to its founding sisters and to the nuns who had served in the Sault for many years. In her reminiscences, Sr. Ste. Constance says, "I will not speak of the scene of our departure; there would be too many sad things to say. For my part, I have never made a greater sacrifice, this mission where we worked so hard, where we had so many conversions, where the people held the sisters in so high esteem ...."

The ladies of the auxiliary presented gifts to Mother Superior Sr. St. Josephat and Sr. Ste. Constance and wrote to thank them: "We have always found you a true friend and your ever willingness to help us in all our undertakings has made them the success they have been. Your cheerful and helpful ways will be missed as we press on in our work .... We wish you both success and God's blessing."[37]

One of the priests, writing from Bishop's House in North Bay to Sr. Ste. Constance, told her, "The hospital is so changed that actually I only made one visit there and had not the heart to go back the second time. Even the nurses that I knew are all gone now, so its charms have vanished for poor me." He closed by saying, "I can assure you I often think with pleasure of the old days when we were happy and when the people of the Sault were happy and we might all be very happy still had things been left as they were."[38] It was the end of an era.

But most endings are also beginnings, and on August 9, 1926, just as had happened twenty-eight years earlier, a group of Grey Sisters arrived in the Sault by train from Ottawa to take on the enormous task of running the hospital. This time there were four — Srs. St. Edith, St. Patricia, Margaret Mary, and Mary Dorothea. They were cordially welcomed by Srs. St. Josephat, St. Urban, St. Blandine, St. Francis Teresa, Ste. Catherine, and St. Fidele. The next day, the Grey Nuns of the Cross left on the noon train "and stern reality began for the Sisters of the Immaculate Conception."[39]

Sisters St. Edith, St. Patricia, and Margaret Mary took on the supervision of the office, kitchen, and operating room, and Sr. Mary Dorothea was named mother superior. She was already very familiar with the hospital, having founded the school of nursing in 1908 and worked at the hospital until 1921. Mary Dorothea, born Eleanor O'Driscoll and raised in Pembroke, had entered the order in 1898 and had taken her nurse's training at her orders' hospital in Ottawa. She administered the General Hospital until 1935 and in later years travelled through Sault Ste. Marie many times on her way to the Grey Sisters' hospitals in Lestock and Esterhazy, Saskatchewan. Her nephew Lawrence O'Driscoll, some years later, was a General Hospital employee and then a member of the hospital's advisory board.

In anticipation of the change of ownership, the local architectural firm of Findlay & Foulis had conducted a valuation of the hospital in 1924. They valued the building and land at $236,000 (building $206,000, land $30,000) and the replacement value of the building only at $315,000.

There were fifty patients in the hospital, $270 in the treasury, and good provisions in the larder and pharmacy. The only debt was a mortgage of $77,000. There were twenty doctors on staff: J.R. McLean, J.R. McRae, A.S. McCaig, S.E. Flemming, J.P. Keith, the Gimbys (father W.E. and son J.E.), A.A. Shephard, J.H. Duncan (x-ray), A. Sinclair Sr., B. Hamilton, W.H. Dudley, C.A. DeSorcey, W.H. Leahy, R.T. Lane, R.F. Cain, S. Casselman, I.M. Lloyd, M. Lowe, and E. Spratt (pathology).

Seventeen young ladies were currently in nurses' training, and there were three graduate nurses on staff as well as sixteen others who were listed as domestics (twelve women and four men).

"For days the sisters laboured untiringly," their Annals read, "and often far into the night, but God was with them and He crowned their efforts with success, for before the month's end everything had been well organized and the confidence and affection of the household won."[40]

In September, they began to buy the livestock that would carry them through the winter, "eight geese, three ducks and a cow," then, "two more cows and a calf, the latter answered to the name Violet."[41]

On October 8, the Annals note a trip of two of the sisters "to the American Soo to shop, but they returned convinced that the Canadian sales were equally advantageous."

Portrait

A Well-Stocked Hospital Pharmacy in 1926

There are thirty-seven drugs and medicinals listed in this pharmacy inventory from the hospital in 1926. Seventy years later in 1998, the Sault Area Hospitals' pharmacy lists about 1,200 items in its formulary.

Morphine* and Atropine*	pre-operative injection
Adrenaline*	injection to treat allergic reaction
Aseptic Ergot	injection to treat post-partum hemorrhage
Chloroform (3 doz. 1 lb. bottles)	anaesthetic
Acetophen (25,000 tablets)	pain and fever reduction
Phenacetine Compound (1,000 tablets)	
Syrup of White Pine (1 gallon)	cough medicine
Syrup Cocillana (1 1/2 gallon)	
Iron Arsenate	treatment of anaemia
Beef, Iron & Wine (1 gallon)	tonic
Syrup of Phosphate, Iron,	
Quinine, and Strychnine (1 gallon)	tonic
Syrup of Ferric Phosphate Compound	tonic
Wampole's Cod Liver Oil (1 gallon)	source of Vitamin D
Camphor & Oil for Hypo	liniment
Betuline Liniment (1/2 gallon)	
Soda Phosphate (3 lbs.)	saline purgative
Milk of Magnesia* (1 gallon)	laxative
Cascara Aromatic* (1 gallon)	
Magnolax* (1 gallon)	
Magnesium Citrate*	
Taka Diastase (1/2 gallon)	digestive aid
Digestive Hypophosphate (1 gallon)	

Hypophos Compound (1 gallon)

Ophthalmic ointment	eye ointment for relief from allergies
Adrenalin ointment	
Yellow Oxide ointment	antibacterial eye ointment
BFI Powder	antiseptic
Scarlet Red Ointment	ointment to promote healing of burns, etc.
Tincture of Iodine	disinfectant
Gentian Compound (1 gallon)	anti-fungal for topical use
Hydrogen Peroxide* (3 gallons)	antiseptic for cleansing wounds

Digitalone	heart drug
Aromatic Red Elixir (1/4 gallon)	flavoured liquid used to dissolve medicinals
Aromatic Spirits of Ammonia (1/2 gallon)	smelling salts
Liquid Peptone (1 gallon)	reagent solution
Three Bromides	chemical reagent

Rye (10 gallons)
Brandy (2 gallons)
Champagne (3 bottles)
Gin (4 bottles)
Wine (4 gallons)

*items still used

Twenty Years of Calm

The most peaceful and stable decades in the General Hospital's hundred-year history were the 1930s and 1940s. This is not to say that the work was easy. But the hospital's records leave a sense that there was a common understanding among the community, staff, doctors, and patients about what the hospital could provide. Operating funds, while never assured, let alone lavish, were adequate to pay the bills. It was an extended moment of calm before the pressures of medical technology, funding shortfalls, job specialization, and community expectations exploded on to the hospital world. Ironically, the tumultuous years of the Great Depression and the Second World War were the years of greatest calm for the General Hospital.

Money flowed out for the normal day-to-day expenses of running an institution: food, drugs and medical supplies, utilities, taxes and insurance, laundry, linen and furnishings, office expenses, and maintenance. Apart from x-ray expenses, there were no large outlays to purchase or maintain the expensive medical equipment and supplies that are commonplace today. In 1935 the General reported to the Ministry of Health a workforce of thirteen student nurses, who received room and board and $5 per month; six laundry workers (room and board and $7 per month); one janitor (room and board and $30 per month); a millwright (room and board and $40 per month); and an engineer for the laundry equipment ($2 per day). There were from ten to fifteen sisters working at the hospital, and for most of the staff in 1935, the hospital was also their home. By the late 1940s, the paid staff was expanding to include nurses and nursing school staff, bookkeepers, orderlies, lab assistants, and a pharmacist. By 1952, there was a paid staff of ninety-two.

Funding was reasonably adequate to handle day-to-day expenses. The Public Hospitals Act had been passed in 1931, and by 1934 the provincial government was paying a total of almost $2,000,000 to 162 hospitals, while the municipalities paid $3,700,000. Revenue came in from paying patients, the province, the city, Workmen's Compensation, local corporations for treatment of their workers, the Department of Indian Affairs, and from outpatient testing (x-rays, lab tests, etc.). As Sr. Mary Dorothea said in her 1932 report, "During this period of general depression, the Hospital like the individual is suffering but in spite of this fact, the current debts are met ...."

The Ministry of Health's 1934 hospital spreadsheet

showed the General's operating cost for the year at $30,790, income at $25,505, and a mortgage of $65,000 which was balanced somewhat by funds held in reserve.

The sisters often referred to the hospital as the house ("At present there are 60 patients in the house") and in many ways, the sisters, the staff who boarded, and the patients (some of whom were patients for weeks) were like a sprawling family — "Fr. Mulligan favored us by moving pictures from his own camera," and "Entertainment held in the Surgical Ward so that the patients could profit," report the *Annals*.[42]

Like a self-sufficient manor house, the hospital produced most of its own food. The *Annals* report "1,000 raspberry bushes were planted, also two dozen of blackberry, some crabapple and pear trees." Later, "The men are storing away the garden produce and the sisters are still enjoying their boat tours [they had a small rowboat to use on the river at their doorstep] although the weather is getting a little chilly .... Our jam cellar is well filled with jams and jelly made by the sisters during the summer and we expect that after the fruit shower given by the Ladies that we will have enough for the winter .... Sr. Superior has purchased three young pigs. We will certainly be living high this winter."[43]

The *Annals* report the daily rhythm of the hospital world — priests visiting, new sisters arriving to take up the work, celebrations of special days, and details of Auxiliary fundraising events. They note the marriage of "Dr. H.E. Spratt, pathologist of the institution [to] Miss Mae Hacket, trained nurse of this city. They left on the noon train for Eastern points." The growth of the entertainment industry was visible even in the hospital — "Four patients on Second Floor agreed to pay the rent of a radio for one month. The 'Victor' is installed and not only

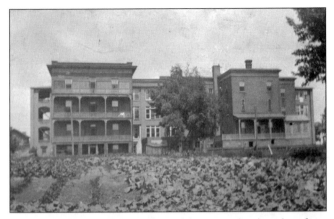

The hospital's own gardens, along with community donations from the annual fruit shower, provided the bulk of the food for patients, sisters, staff, and students. The early nuns also kept cows and chickens. **Courtesy *The Sault Star***

furnishes music but acts as a palliative treatment in helping the sick to recover cheerfully."[44]

Events of the city and the world are observed — the abdication of Edward VIII (the Prince of Wales), the Sault's preparations for war — as well as the sisters' breaks in routine — picnics with the rowboat, trips to camps at Achigan Lake and Gros Cap, skating parties with the Sisters of St. Joseph, and occasional movies. One continuing story details the second youth of one of the city's doctors. In the spring of 1941, the sisters were surprised to hear that the doctor had married a young lady in Beverly Hills, California. Several weeks later, he arrived home "with his charming young wife, bringing her to the hospital to see and meet the Sisters first. She presented Sister Superior with the 'Ave Maria' by Guonod in fantasy style by Walt Disney." Several weeks later the young wife called again at the hospital to take Sister Superior to see the magnificent home they had purchased at the top of Pim Hill, the estate of a former judge. Sister pronounced the grounds beautiful but neglected and the house sadly in need of repair. About a month later, the *Annals* note that the doctor was "brought in by ambulance in an unconscious condition."[45] He recovered and continued his practice but never merited another mention in the hospital record.

There was continued goodwill toward the hospital on the part of the Sault's largest employer, Algoma Steel, and Sir James Dunn was personally acquainted with the sisters. In 1951 he offered his private plane to fly a group of sisters up to Wawa to inspect the new Lady Dunn Hospital. Throughout the year, the Ladies' Auxiliary and the Nurses' Alumnae held fruit showers, shamrock sales, linen showers, tag days, euchre parties, garden parties, and draws to raise money for the hospital, all well attended and generously supported. The General was part of the social rhythm of the community.

But the *Annals* also chronicle the increasing complexity of the hospital world and foreshadow the directions it would take in later decades. Nurses' stations were set up in the wards in 1942; new dishwashers, new typewriters, crowded conditions in the nursery, the need for a larger pediatric ward, in-patient numbers of 100 when the usual number was 40, the hiring of a professional dietitian, the purchase of a hemoglobumeter for the lab — ("It was necessary to procure one as we were greatly criticized by some doctors for how we took hemoglobins"[46]) — were just a few of the changes during these two decades.

Portrait

Christmas at the Hospital

This is the entry in the Sisters' Annals *for Christmas 1929.*

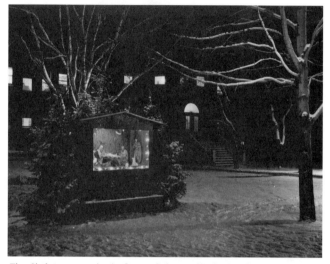

The Christmas creche in front of the medical wing front door.

Dear old Christmas dawned once more and everything was grandiose in the spiritual as well as the temporal line. The Sisters and Nurses attended midnight Mass at the parish church and were very much impressed by the beautiful singing and sweet music. There were four masses in the hospital chapel, accompanied by the sweet strains of the Christmas carols. Dame Flora graced the feast with the abundance of her garden. The profusion, variety and hue of the cut flowers and seasonal plants gave the chapel the appearance of a veritable flower garden. The beautifully trimmed trees, loaded with presents, the bright decorations of green, red and gold together with the chatter of the little ones crowing over their presents, and the merry laughter of the nurses gave a festive tone to the whole scene. The night supervisor, Miss Goatby, dressed as Santa Claus drew the gifts while the dean, Dr. McLean, and his assistants Drs. McRae, McCaig and Sabetta, the latter all the way from sunny Italy, sat around smiling and applauding.

The surgery was so important that Christmas Day was not exempt. There were two operations, one at 10 a.m. and the other at 3:30 p.m. The Sisters also had a pretty little Christmas tree set up in the Community [their dormitory area] by one of the nurses. Sr. Margaret Mary drew the presents, all the while having an eye on her own. The gifts were many and the flowers for the chapel were given by the alumnae, pupils and graduate nurses and friends. The sumptuous dinner was served at 12 a.m. to which everyone did justice.

Rev. Father Crowley P.P. gave benediction of the Blessed Sacrament at 4 p.m., after which all proceeded to the Community to receive his blessing. Letters came pouring in, also cards of good wishes. Among the number, one is worthy of note. "To dear Sr. Mary Dorothea, Superior, with love and our dear Sisters, Christmas greetings with love. May the New Year come to you laden with God's choicest blessings. Mother Kirby."

Supper was served at the usual hour, after which recreation was spent very pleasantly talking over the events of the day, while examining the pretty Christmas cards and from time to time listening to the catchy airs of the victrola. At 8:30 all tendered a vote of thanks to the worthy Superior, followed by night prayer, after which the Sisters withdrew and silence reigned supreme.

The entry for New Year's Day reads, "New Year's was celebrated with all religious ceremony available. The day was very quiet and uneventful. There were no Community visitors. The outlook for the future was quite bright."

Accommodating a Booming City
Accommodating a Booming City

The postwar decades promised to be boom years for Ontario. In Sault Ste. Marie, Algoma Steel boomed, the population boomed and the General Hospital, which entered the 1950s with only ninety-six beds, seemed about ready to burst.

The solution was the same in the Sault as it was all over Ontario — build new hospitals. The provincial and federal governments had by this time agreed to cost-share in order to fund hospital construction, a collaborative arrangement which has been the foundation for all subsequent health policy in Canada. From 1954 to 1971 the number of hospital beds in Ontario more than doubled — from 22,000 to 52,000. The General and Plummer Hospitals both added extensive new wings in the 1950s and 1960s, almost quadrupling the number of beds — from 163 to approximately 600! On both occasions they planned jointly and for the 1963 expansion they also fundraised together. At the General, the expansion took place in two phases — the New Pavilion (B Wing) in 1954 and the new hospital (A and Y Wings) in 1963.

Plans for the New Pavilion were announced in November 1951 on the same day that the Plummer announced its own expansion plans. The wing was built just off the old hospital's southwest corner, the two parts being connected on each floor by a narrow hallway running along the north face of the addition. These hallways are now long narrow rooms at the Queen St. end of each B Wing floor.

Algoma Steel Corporation, the Sault's major employer, took a leading role in the fundraising campaign for both hospitals and produced a glossy booklet with a foreword signed by Sir James Dunn. The booklet placed the area's population at 65 000 and estimated that the new hospital bed counts would be 180 for the General (from 96) and 78 for the Plummer (from 67), an enormous 70 per cent increase. "Strained out of all proportion," the booklet states, "[the hospitals] are today alarmingly inadequate to meet the demands made upon them."

The General conducted an extensive fundraising campaign. Room plaques were prepared for every donor of $500 or more and these plaques can still be seen on some of the B Wing doors. In all, the community donated $180,000.

Construction began in September 1952 while G.A. McGuire was chair of the Advisory Board and Sr. Mary Augustine was administrator. The Toronto firm of Harold J. Smith served as architects and the contractor was the local firm of Jannison & Scott. The cornerstone was laid in September 1953 in a small ceremony presided over by Msgr. Crowley. One *Sault Star* account mentions an innovative construction technique: no rivets were used in the steel beams, all conections being welded. In the end the project cost $1,300,000 and added eighty-eight beds and thirty-three bassinettes to the hospital.

October 28, 1954, was the grand opening day. Patients gained three new units: private rooms on the first floor, Pediatrics on the second and Obstetrics on the third, with a coffee shop for visitors in the basement. The sisters gained a new twenty-six room residence on the fourth floor and a beautiful community room overlooking the river. In the old hospital, their residence had been a large dormitory and several sisters recall their delight at these new upscale accomodations. Staff gained several new services, including two small cafeterias on the ground floor, a laundry and an oxygen preparation area. The wing was heated with a coal-burning furnace.

A special *Sault Star* tabloid commemorating the opening brings congratulations from local suppliers — Cochrane Dunlop Hardware, Algoma Bakery, Mayfair Bakery, J. McLeod & Sons, Soo Mill & Lumber, Lyons Fuel, Taylor Bros, Vic Haft Home Furnishings, J.C. Pinch Stores — some gone but many still in business forty-five years later.

Planning began almost immediately for the second stage of expansion: a completely new central wing and demolition of the old hospital. Introducing these plans to the community in 1960, administrator Sr. Teresa Agatha commented that the operation of the General Hospital was "big business — the business of human life."

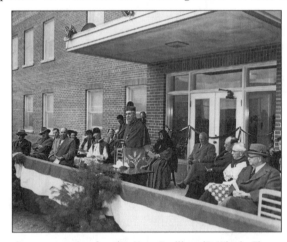

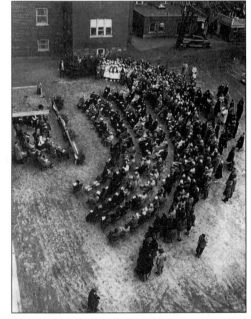

Opening ceremonies for the New Pavilion (B Wing). The ceremonies took place on the east side of the wing. The old hospital is visible at the top of the picture on the right. The close-up photo shows (left to right) Mayor Herb Smale (hatless), Msgr. Crowley, Bishop R. Dignan (speaking), Superior General Mary Dorothy, Algoma Steel president David S. Holbrook, Msgr. J. O'Leary, and MPP Harry Lyons.

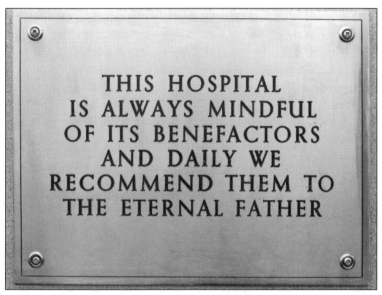

THIS HOSPITAL
IS ALWAYS MINDFUL
OF ITS BENEFACTORS
AND DAILY WE
RECOMMEND THEM TO
THE ETERNAL FATHER

This plaque in the B Wing elevator commemorates the donations to the New Pavilion.

Since funding for hospital redevelopment was now controlled by the Ontario Hospital Services Commission (OHSC), the Plummer and General, of necessity, prepared their plans jointly. Extensive correspondence passed between the hospital and the OHSC and the hospital was required to show that its planning was sound, its figures accurate and its fundraising hopes secure.

The total expansion cost for both hospitals was estimated at $6,000,000: $2,000,000 for a new west wing at the Plummer and $4,000,000 for new centre and south wings at the General. The result would be 327 beds at the General (from 201) and 288 beds at the Plummer (from 165). The province put in half the funds, while the city agreed to contribute $1,750,000 and the townships of Korah and Tarantorus $100,000 each. The Grey Sisters agreed to hold a twenty-year $1,000,000 mortgage in addition to an existing hospital debt of $230,500. This left $800,000 to be fundraised from the community ($400,000 for each hospital) and Lawrence Brown, Assistant to the President at Algoma Steel, was named to head up the Joint Hospitals Committee. Algoma Steel contributed $200,000 to the campaign and with hard work it was able to surpass its goal.

The project was essentially an opportunity to design a new hospital and much credit must go to administrator Sr. Teresa Agatha for overseeing the development of a beautiful and efficient hospital which is admirably standing the test of time. Several features were considered innovative: the Emergency department was placed so as to be immediately accessible to lab and x-ray; the patient units were designed to have double corridors with the nursing station positioned in the centre; canopied entrances were constructed at the front door and at Emergency; and for visitors, the front lobby, parking lot entrance, elevators, and cafeteria were positioned in close proximity.

New patient units included Intensive Care, Psychiatry, and Long Term Care and there was also an extensive rehabilitation facility. A stunning chapel with walls of stained glass windows juts out at the front of the hospital and the sisters gained additional space and a new private chapel on the Y Wing fourth floor.

The Sudbury firm of Fabbro and Townend were the architects and Robertson Yates from Hamilton was the contractor. Steel was used extensively in the construction, with over eighty per cent being supplied by Algoma Steel.

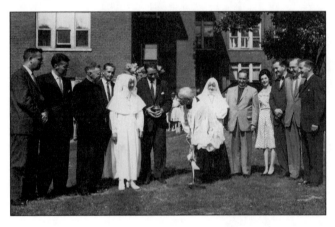

Breaking the sod for the new hospital in 1961. Left to right are Henry Lang, James McIntyre, Rev. C. Adams, Dr. A. Scott, Sr. Teresa Agatha, L. Fabbro, Msgr. J. O'Leary, Sr. Mary Camillus, Rev. F. Nock, Peggy Keenan, A. Townend, J. Bailey, Laurence Brown.

The new hospital was built directly behind the old one and connected to the B Wing. On completion, the furnishings and equipment were transferred to the new building. Items not needed were sold at auction by the Auxiliary and the patients were moved in. Then the old 1898 building with its two additions, the Medical Wing and the Gibson Wing, fell to the wrecker's ball. The spacious front lawn of the present hospital covers over the foundations of the old buildings and the new hospital and parking lot occupy

the site of the sisters' old gardens and orchard, their skating rink and the outbuildings where they had kept, among other animals, the cow which "answered to the name of Violet."

The opening ceremonies were held November 7, 1963, chaired by Advisory Board president Henry Lang. Msgr. O'Leary presided, Lawrence Brown gave the address and the St. Mary's Glee Club sang.

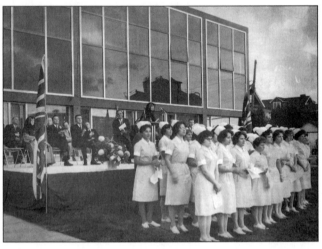

Opening ceremonies for the new hospital, just outside the new cafeteria. Sr. Teresa Agatha is speaking and to her immediate right are Dr. William Hutchinson, James McIntyre, and Laurence Brown. Students from St. Mary's School of Nursing are in front of the stage.

Did anyone attending the ceremonies realize the importance of the new player who had entered the hospital arena? From the 1960s forward, the voice of the provincial (and federal) governments joined the traditional voices of the community, the physicians, and the city fathers in hospital decisionmaking. Health care was becoming enormously expensive — by 1990 it consumed one third of the Ontario budget. The provincial government was now paying the piper and quite rightly it wanted a say in calling the tune. Increasingly the government began to ask all healthcare providers in each community to plan and work together and in 1993, thirty years after their last great expansions, the Plummer and General in Sault Ste. Marie were among the first hospitals to do just that.

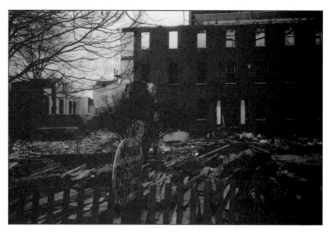

The end of an era, the old building is demolished and the new hospital appears behind it.

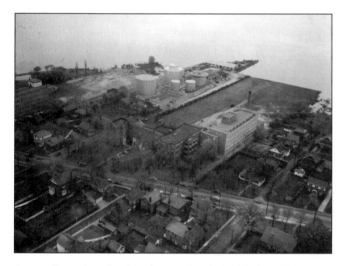

An excellent view showing the new hospital with the old hospital still standing. The Plummer Hospital is visible at the left. The Doctors Building has yet to be built between the two hospitals.

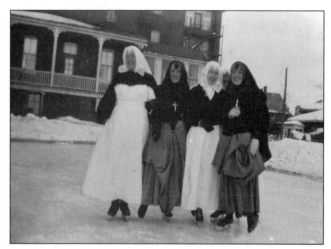

Dr. Charles Eaid, who grew up on Gordon Street beside the hospital, remembers there always being a skating rink behind the hospital. Here Srs. Mary Melanie, Mary Blanche, Anthony of Padua, Teresa Agatha, and Rita Kennedy (left to right) enjoy some leisure time.

Portrait

A Diamond Jubilee: Celebrating Sixty Years

Three days of celebrations marked the 60th anniversary of the General Hospital and the 50th anniversary of the St. Mary's School of Nursing in 1958. The festivities were arranged for June 18–20, 1958, to coincide with the nursing graduation ceremonies, and nursing school alumni were invited for a grand reunion as well.

Wednesday, June 18, was a day for the nursing grads. Other special guests for the day were St. Mary's alumni, who were invited for a reunion weekend, priests from all parts of the diocese, and twenty-one Grey Sisters who came from other hospitals.

The second day began with mass at the hospital chapel celebrated by Msgr. T.J. Crowley. A community tea was held in the afternoon, and the alumni gathered for dinner at the Golden Steer. In the evening, the Sault Concert Band gave a concert on the hospital grounds.

On the closing day, Msgr. J.J. O'Leary celebrated the morning mass, and W.J. Smith, bishop of Pembroke, officiated at an afternoon ceremony held to recognize long-serving employees. Henry Lang, chair of the hospital's advisory board, also spoke. The longest-serving employee was radiologist Dr. J.B. Symington. The nursing students entertained in the evening at a variety show at St. Ignatius Hall.

It was an occasion of great joy and pride and was a prelude to the great expansion of the 1960s.

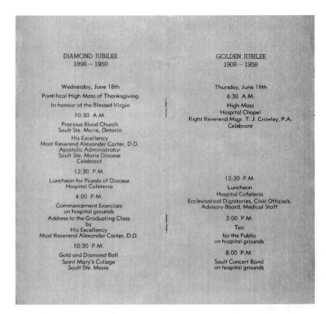

The Jubilee program.

Better Together

What might seem obvious and simple in retrospect was, at the time, difficult and painful to achieve. Today, the General Hospital and its sister hospital the Plummer — which sit side by side on Queen Street — operate in a partnership that has been a unique development among hospitals in Ontario. The partnership, called Sault Area Hospitals, allows the General and Plummer to maintain their own boards of directors, thus preserving their own mission and values, but to reap the benefits that come from planning and working in concert. But if the marriage is a success, the courtship was long and tumultuous.

At the grassroots level there was always loyalty to one's own institution and also a competitive rivalry. But there was also, always, a quiet cooperation between the two hospital staffs. Dr. Alex Sinclair recalls the practice of ordering the even-numbered sizes of expensive Kuntscher nails — used in orthopedic surgery — for one hospital and the odd sizes for the other. The surgeon would simply request a nail from the other hospital if it was necessary. Expensive traction equipment was shared, as were pharmacy supplies. The nursing schools cooperated, having some of their lectures delivered jointly. The auxiliaries attended conferences together and gave some teas jointly. Professional counterparts invited each other to attend continuing education sessions. But at the institutional level, it was a case of Macy's and Gimbel's. Neither would tell the other its plans, but there was plenty of looking across the street to see what "they" were doing. One physician recalls that virtually the same minutes could have been taken at the meetings of the two medical advisory committees.

The turning point was 1963, the year both hospitals completed substantial building programs. It was both the zenith of competition and the beginning of institutional cooperation, since the fundraising for these expansions had been conducted jointly. Finally, thirty years later, in 1993, the General and Plummer had travelled far enough down the same pathway that they were able to hire a common president and CEO, Manu Malkani.

Through the 1960s, there were signals that competition between the hospitals no longer made sense. Medical equipment was becoming staggeringly expensive. The Ministry of Health was tightening its purse strings. The community was beginning to demand a fully staffed twenty-four hour Emergency department.

Tentative overtures were made in 1966 with the formation of a Joint Hospital Advisory Committee, which recommended that a number of services be consolidated. This initiative received a boost when the schools of nursing were moved out of both hospitals in 1970 and the Plummer nurses' residence became available. In a chain reaction, the Plummer Nurses' Residence became vacant; the General's psychiatric unit moved into the building, which was renamed River View Centre; and obstetrical services began to consolidate at the General in the former psychiatric area. A sophisticated and expensive Neonatal Intensive Care Unit was developed at one hospital only, the General, and designed to serve the entire community. This much rationalization was successfully complete by 1981, the year of the opening of the NICU. At the same time, the two hospital labs began to develop areas of specialization, and a pneumatic tube was installed to carry products routinely between the labs.

In the meantime, progress on fuller institutional cooperation was more difficult. At the Ministry of Health's request in 1980, the District Health Council commissioned Woods Gordon Management Consultants to complete a role study for the two hospitals. The final report recommended amalgamation, a concept unacceptable to either hospital board. Instead, the hospitals formed a Coordination of Institutional Services Committee to attempt to hammer out a rationalization agreement themselves. The General Hospital's representatives were CEO Jerry Betik; board chairs Bill Struk, followed by Dr. Lou Lukenda; Chief of Staff Dr. Pat O'Neill; Sr. Marguerite Hennessy; and Charles Vaillancourt. This committee laboured for almost four years and finally signed a comprehensive rationalization agreement on February 28, 1986. In addition to dividing medical specialties between the

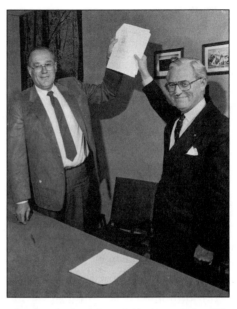

Dr. Lou Lukenda, General board chair, and Franklin Prouse, Plummer board chair, sign the 1986 rationalization agreement between the two hospitals. **Courtesy *The Sault Star***

two hospitals, the report recommended construction of a jointly administered Central Service Unit (CSU) to be located on property between the two hospitals. The CSU would house an Emergency unit, lab, ambulatory care clinics, most support services and a diagnostic imaging unit containing the proposed CT scanner and other equipment that was obviously too expensive to be duplicated.

The Ministry refused to give approval or funding to the CSU concept, saying in 1989 that the two hospitals along with the Group Health Centre and other local health providers should "explore options and opportunities for coordination and integration of the health system in Sault Ste. Marie." Once again, the province was telling the Sault hospitals that they must move closer together, if not via a merger as had been suggested in 1980, then through some form of partnership that would truly attack the problem of duplication of services at the two hospitals.

And so, through 1991 and 1992, a group of eleven people struggled to work out an agreement acceptable to the two hospital boards, the Group Health Centre, the Grey Sisters, the Ministry of Health, and the community. The group was known as Health Horizons (Algoma) Inc. and was made up of three board members from each hospital and the Group Health Centre, one Grey Sister, and one physician. Since it was necessary to ensure that the General's Catholic philosophy would be protected, the group chose as its facilitator, Sr. Melanie di Pietro, a sister and a lawyer cognizant of canon law. After only five months of full-scale negotiations, Sr. Melanie and the group were able to achieve a first in Ontario — a partnership between a Catholic and public hospital. In June 1992 the two hospital boards approved the model — a common CEO and management team, a common chief of staff, and one Medical Advisory Committee, with all physicians having privileges at both hospitals. Each hospital would maintain its own board of directors. The boards would plan and work together by means of the Joint Service Committee composed of the executive of the two boards.

At the hospitals' first joint annual meeting, Minister of Health Ruth Grier congratulated the hospital boards for having "achieved a unique feat by demonstrating how two hospitals can work together and make profound changes without sacrificing the mission, values, and traditions of either organization."[47]

The primary objective of the partnership was to enhance patient services by eliminating duplication and to that end, almost all departments and services have been consolidated. The most visible achievement has been the 1997 consolidation of Emergency to one department, located at the General Hospital.

In 1996, the two hospitals adopted the partnership name Sault Area Hospitals. In 1998, following a formal evaluation of the first four years of the partnership, the hospitals agreed to extend the relationship indefinitely. Both are confident that they are best serving the health needs of the community by working together.

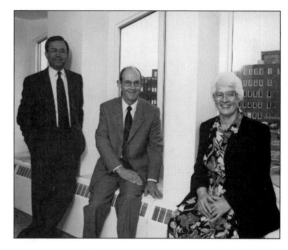

Manu Malkani (left) CEO of Sault Area Hospitals, with General board chair Michael Mingay and vice chair Sr. Diane Carty. The Plummer Hospital, partner to the General, is visible through the window.

The Caregivers

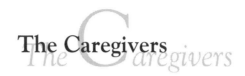

The hospital ... is peculiarly characteristic of our society.
Within the walls of a single building, high technology, bureaucracy, and professionalism
are juxtaposed with the most fundamental and unchanging
of human experiences — birth, death, pain.

Charles Rosenberg in *The Care of Strangers*

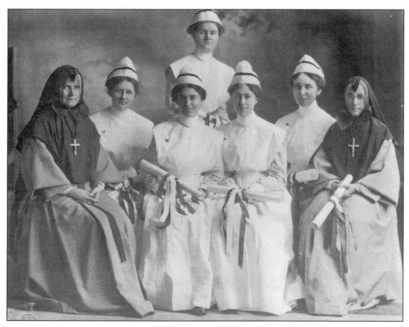

1915 graduation ceremonies for the St. Mary's School of Nursing. Sr. Mary
Dorothea, whose association with the General spanned two orders and four
decades, is at the left, with Mary Gleason, Veronica Lavigne, Anne Mary Sheedy,
Mary Delaney, Sr. Mary Helen, and Laura O'Connor (back).

Sault Ste. Marie Hospital Core Values

Justice is found when we deal uprightly with absolute fairness.

Hospitality
Spirituality
Vision
Justice
Sacredness of Life

The Doctors

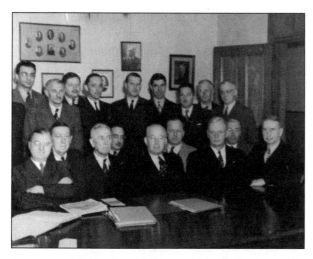

A meeting of the medical board, around 1947. Front row, l to r: Drs. Roberts, N.F.W. Graham, S.E. Flemming, C.H. Shaver, E. Spratt, J.D. Sprague, E. Gimby, T.R. Heath, A. Sinclair. Back row, l to r: Drs. E.J.M. Greco, J.B. Symington, I. Smith, E.S. Pentland, C.H. Greig, T.A. Breton, B.W. Casselman, J. Johnston, R.F. Cain. Photos of Sault doctors who had died are behind them on the wall.

The first of the modern, scientifically trained group of doctors to establish a practice in Sault Ste. Marie was Dr. Thomas Simpson. Simpson had married W.H. Plummer's sister Helen while he was engaged as company physician in Bruce Mines. Relocating to the Sault when Bruce Mines' fortunes waned, he set up his office at the corner of Albert and East Streets, still — in the 1990s — a popular location for doctors' offices. By 1872 Simpson and his wife had moved to Montreal where he became a friend and colleague of Sir William Osler, still revered as one of Canada's most distinguished physicians, and among other accomplishments, the author of the first modern medical textbook, *The Principles and Practice of Medicine*. It was because of this family connection that Osler treated Maria Plummer during her final illness.

Dr. J.A. Reid came next, again via Bruce Mines. There he married Annie Marks, whose younger sister Jennie would become the wife of the man known as the father of the General Hospital, Dr. Robert Gibson. The Reids came to the Sault in 1880, and until his death in 1902, Reid served as CPR physician and physician to the Garden River Band.

During the 1890s, as the economic fortunes of the Sault rose, four more university-educated physicians arrived. The most famous was Gibson, who had previously been a CPR physician in Chapleau. The others were Drs. A.S. McCaig, coroner and respected Medical Officer of Health; S.E. Flemming, Gaol Surgeon, and J.R. McLean, Algoma Steel Physician.

These men were all university trained (Toronto and McGill) and they all needed a hospital to complement the style of medicine they had learned. The four of them cooperatively took on medical responsibilities at the new General Hospital.

They formally organized in March 1901 as the medical staff of the General Hospital and the minutes of their meetings contain something of all aspects of hospital administration. They deliberated on what amount should be charged to the Clergue industries — the "Allied Companies" — for prepaid employee hospital care, finally deciding on $250 per year per bed, an arrangement to exclude, "premeditated medical and surgical cases, together with funeral cases."[48] They took on the power of deciding which new physicians would be allowed to practise in the hospital, and they responded to a written application to the hospital in 1904 by saying that there were at present no medical vacancies. In an effort to raise the hospital's profile and its fundraising abilities, they invited town council to send a delegation to tour the hospital, and they deliberated making presentations to both the Sault and Steelton town councils. In the final recorded minutes of November 1908, the Medical Board agreed to take on the task of lecturing the students of the newly created St. Mary's School of Nursing.

As the Sault continued to industrialize these early physicians were joined by Drs. William Edwin Gimby and his brother John H. Gimby, who also served as mayor for two years; Allan A. Shephard, John R. McRae; James McLurg; Thomas McQuaid; John P. Keith; and Simon Casselman, physician to Algoma Steel and Spanish River Pulp & Paper (the forerunner to E.B. Eddy). The alma mater for all but one was the University of Toronto.

In 1909 this group was joined by a man who would devote forty-six years to his adopted community as physician, member of city council, and a driving force behind the creation of the House of Refuge. Dr. Alexander Sinclair was born in Kilsyth (near Owen Sound) Ontario, and was a U of T graduate. His extensive education makes him stand out — like Gibson, Sinclair took post-graduate surgical training in Britain. In 1911 he organized the town's Medical Society and served as its first president. Sinclair's lifelong medical interest was the thyroid, specifically the breakthrough research on goitre.

By the 1920s these early physicians had been joined by Drs. George D. Fripp; Benson Hamilton possibly the first Sault physician to specialize in eye, ear, nose, and throat medicine; Robert T. Lane; Charles A. DeSorcey; Isaac Cohen; Joseph E. Gimby, son of Dr. W.E. Gimby, and John H. Duncan. Duncan was raised in Sault Ste. Marie while his father was pastor of St. Andrew's Presbyterian (now United) Church. He commenced practice in Bruce Mines and came to Sault Ste. Marie after Dr. Gibson's death to continue his hospital x-ray work. Following Dr. Duncan in the early 1920s were Drs. I.M. Lloyd, W.H. Dudley, John McDonald, Robert F. Cain, Nelson F.W. Graham, Hugh W. Johnston, and W.H. Leahy. Again, almost all were U of T graduates.

The General's medical staff reconstituted itself in 1921, and there is a complete record of its meetings from that date until 1941. At various times, it called itself the Medical Staff, Medical Board, and finally the Hospital Board. The position of president became today's twin positions of Chief of Staff and President of Medical Staff; however, the concept of a full Medical Advisory Committee did not evolve until the growth of specialization following the Second World War. A similar board functioned at the Plummer Hospital, and there was also a city-wide Medical Society. The meeting format was generally a discussion of hospital statistics from the previous month, debate over outstanding issues of the day, and presentation of an interesting case. In the early years, patient names were used and, on occasion, the patient himself was brought to the meeting. "The patient [with Buerger's Disease] was examined by the members present and a full discussion followed."[49] The senior Dr. Sinclair reminisced at his retirement that, in those days, the physicians wore black tie to their monthly meetings.

Part of the board's reason for existence was to allow the hospital to comply with the standards of the American College of Surgeons, which had taken on a form of hospital accreditation. To this end, physicians were required to keep detailed patient charts and histories, and, at almost every meeting, there is a reminder that physicians are falling behind in this area and must be diligent. Finally a Record Committee was formed to oversee chart completion, and in 1934 the services of a stenographer were provided.

The minutes show a profession trying to carve out a niche for itself within a new style of institution. Many of the issues they grappled with are still with us today. There are repeated urgings that physicians should focus on diagnosis (both pre- and post-op); they discussed all aspects of patient care, including "some discussion as to meals served patients not being appropriate to patient needs and sometimes cold."[50] Physicians repeatedly requested a room to conduct post-mortems and there was general pleasure with the hiring of Dr. Spratt as pathologist. A pathology committee was formed shortly after his arrival and, by 1934, all tissues removed during surgery were required to be sent to the pathologist for examination.

The board often discussed hospital finances. In 1932 they sent a resolution to the Ontario Hospital Association stating that "any reduction in the government grants to hospitals at the present would be inadvisable and would work to the detriment of the

public."[51] Several rounds of correspondence with the Workmen's Compensation Board (WCB) dealt with the issue of who paid ambulance and operating room expenses for WCB cases.

The Second World War was a watershed in the practice of medicine in Canada. With the aid of new wonder drugs like sulfa, then penicillin and other antibiotics, physicians for the first time were able to focus on cure. Advances in surgical techniques originated during the war, the development of intravenous therapy, and the new ability to do blood transfusions made complex surgeries more feasible. Almost routinely, physicians were able to intervene and change the course of a disease.

A large group of family physicians established practices in the Sault during and after the war years, caring for the families of a thriving steel town, and they are held in special esteem for their care and expertise during the joyful, sorrowful, and other momentous occasions of many lives. The photos accompanying this chapter will evoke memories for many who have lived and worked in postwar Sault Ste. Marie.

Also in the postwar period, physicians for the first time began to arrive with post-graduate training in new specialties such as pediatrics, obstetrics, orthopedics, and ophthalmology. Dr. C.H. Greig, a graduate of U of T's new post-graduate surgical program, arrived in 1946 at the direct invitation of Sir James Dunn and took on the position of chief of staff immediately on his arrival, responsible for a medical staff of twenty. He was joined by surgeons Dr. William Hutchinson in 1949 and Dr. Alex Sinclair (son of the city's first Dr. Alex Sinclair) in 1950. Dr. Thomas Black and Dr. William Robertson arrived in 1950 as the city's first obstetrician and pediatrician. In the mid-fifties, three more surgeons, Dr. Kent Armstrong, Dr. Fred Baar, and Dr. William Kelly, began their practices. On into the 1960s the specialty ranks expanded to include Dr. D.K. Newbigging (ear, nose, and throat), Dr. S.A. Shamess and Dr. S. Golesic (ophthalmology), Dr. G. Rundle (internal medicine), Dr. A. Lalonde (thoracic surgery), Dr. P. Kowalyshn (urology), and Dr. Pat Fyfe (orthopedic surgery). In 1966 there were fifty-four physicians on the General's medical staff. By 1976 the number had jumped to ninety-nine.

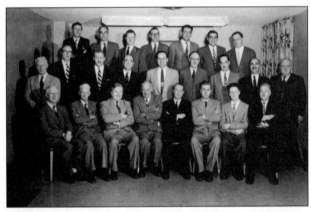

Physicians on staff in the late 1950s. First row, l to r: Drs. H. Johnston, B. Symington, I. Smith, D. Cowan, B. Greco, T. Black, G. Rundle, B. Casselman. Middle row: J. McDonald, K. Armstrong, W. Kelly, W. Robertson, S. Shamess, R. Sparks, C. Shaver, A. Gardi, H. Leahy. Top row: M. West, F. Baar, J. Gibson, C. Eaid, E. Greco, R. Carbon, L. Sagle.

As physicians began to specialize and medicine became increasingly compartmentalized, the General Hospital began to respond with specialized facilities. When the new hospital was opened in 1963, it included units for pediatrics, obstetrics, psychiatry, medicine, surgery, and emergency medicine. In 1968 the hospital opened two more specialty units: coronary care (under the direction of Dr. D. Gould) and intensive care. In 1981 the General opened the neo-natal intensive care unit and in 1991, the palliative care unit.

In the General's centennial year, the chief of staff is Dr. Bruce Skinner, presiding over a medical staff of approximately 130, almost half of whom are specialists, and the General, in partnership with the Plummer Hospital, offers a full range of services supported by these physicians. The medical program includes internal medicine, oncology, dialysis, and cardiology. The surgical program includes vascular, plastic, orthopedic, ear/nose/throat, urological and gynecological surgery. The maternal and child program includes obstetrics, pediatrics, and neonatal intensive care. Mental health and long-term care round out the services.

The St. Mary's School of Nursing

The St. Mary's School of Nursing

The St. Mary's School of Nursing was founded in 1908, ten years after the hospital opened. The opening of the Medical Wing in that year had freed up space in the original building, which could then be used as a student dormitory. The first student was Miss Ivy Reynolds, a young woman who lived on Front Street, "right beside the hospital." In 1958 Sr. Teresa Agatha, retired administrator of the General, related the story of the school's founding to the *Sault Star*. She had been told the story by Sr. Mary Dorothea: "A girl who lived nearby approached her (Mary Dorothea) one morning as she sat on the verandah and in the course of the conversation she told (her) that she wished to become a nurse. At that time there was no training school for nurses connected with the hospital so Sr. Mary Dorothea, being a nurse herself [a graduate of Ottawa General], agreed to tutor her individually. 'Come back tomorrow morning and we'll start a school of nursing,' she said."[52] Thus, without fuss or fanfare, the commonsense and straightforward origins of a school that would proudly graduate over five hundred nurses over the course of sixty-three years.

The concept of training schools attached to hospitals was by this time well established in Ontario, the first being the Mack School, established in 1874, part of the St. Catharines General and Marine Hospital. These schools had twin objectives: to provide a professional nurse's training in the Nightingale tradition and to guarantee a source of unpaid labour for the hospital. The discipline was rigid, the work was hard, the hours were long, and tremendous responsibility was entrusted to students. Upon receiving their diploma, graduate nurses left the hospital — there was no expectation that a hospital would pay staff nurses. Still, nursing became a popular and professionally rewarding profession and it attracted young women of dedication and spirit.

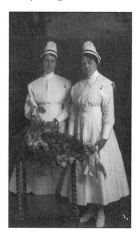

Catherine McGaghran and Mildred Gaston, the St. Mary's graduating class of 1922.

From the beginning, the General's training course was three years long. Sr. Mary Dorothea and the other sisters who were graduate nurses gave instruction in the practicalities of nursing care, including the preparation of diets, hygiene and ventilation, and the actions and uses of medicines. The town's doctors (Gibson, McCaig, Fleming and McLean) lectured on the standards of anatomy, physiology, obstetrics, etc. Most instruction was given at the bedside. Girls entered training one or two at a time and so their first few months were akin to an apprenticeship.

Sr. Teresa Agatha related that, together, Sr. Mary Dorothea and Ivy Reynolds chose the student uniform — floor-length blue-and-white striped cotton shirtwaist, covered with a white apron and worn with starched white collar and cuffs. A local dressmaker sewed the uniforms for $2, and each student received two sets of uniforms per year (plus $4 per month for books, etc.). Over the years, this basic style stayed the same — with shorter and shorter skirts — until it was replaced in 1962 with a simple one-piece dress.

Rules were stringent. Students had to be twenty years old and have an education equal to that required for a public school teaching certificate. They had to have been vaccinated and be able to show a vaccination mark. They needed a certificate of good character from a clergyman and a certificate of good health from a physician. As late as 1954, a *Sault Star* article noted that the nursing course was open to young women "who can give satisfactory evidence of seriousness of purpose and uprightness of character." [53]

It went without question that the students, like the nursing sisters, lived in the hospital. Nursing was looked on as a full-time commitment, much like the position of a governess. Ivy Reynolds remembered working twelve hour days (7 a.m. to 7 p.m.), "and if things were very busy, they might ask us if we would mind working another twelve." Miss Reynolds recalled, "looking after mothers and babies all day and then going to bed in the same room with the babies, getting up to look after feedings during the night. 'If your mother could only see you now,' " was a friend's comment one evening on finding her in bed with an infant on each arm.

Students did the bulk of the hospital work. Miss Reynolds remembered doing "the cleaning, nursing, answering doors and the telephone. The work was entirely different then," she told the *Sault Star*. "In those days everything was poultices. We'd have to go down to the furnace to make linseed poultices." For the first graduation "we moved all the beds out of the big [medical] ward. We scrubbed the floor and brought chairs. Our parents and friends were invited and pretty well filled the room. There were no frills. We just got our diplomas and pins, from Dr. Gibson I think. He was head doctor at that time."

Six girls graduated in the first class. Surprisingly, Ivy Reynolds was the only Saultite. One student, Armenia Brabant, came from Michigan. Mildred Kehoe (probably a niece of J.J. Kehoe) from Wyman, Quebec; Loretta Contway from Pembroke; Jean Scott from Webbwood, and Mary Waters from Fallowfield, near Ottawa, rounded out the class.

Upon graduation, the nurse could try for a job in the growing field of public health or take work as a private-duty nurse. These nurses were independent entrepreneurs who were called into homes at times of sickness either by the family or the doctor. They lived in and were expected to be on duty twenty-four hours a day, with responsibilities for the house as well as the patient. In the early days, standard wages were $5 per week, paid by the family. It was also common for private-duty nurses to work in the hospital, "specialing" patients whose families had hired them. In the 1930s, sixty per cent of Canadian nurses were employed as private-duty nurses, and as late as the

1950s, the General and Plummer kept a registry of grads who were available for private-duty nursing. Student nurses also worked as private-duty nurses to gain experience, their wages going to the hospital. Annie (Gibson) Andrews, a 1913 graduate, remembered going "out on cases" in her final year. Following graduation, Miss Reynolds travelled to Coppercliff, east of Sudbury, where she headed the VON until her retirement.

Graduation was always a special and festive occasion. At the 1916 gradation, seven graduates (again only one from Sault Ste. Marie) received their diplomas. Superior General Duhamel travelled from Ottawa for the occasion, and Dr. McCaig and Dr. Gibson addressed the graduates as did Fr. McMenamin and Rev. Bunbury. Several soloists performed, and the Orpheum orchestra played for the crowd — of about 300!

A milestone in the school's history was the opening of the Gibson Memorial Wing in 1923. This spacious three-storey wing became both residence and classroom for almost forty classes of nursing students. A gracious nurses' parlour and library took up the main floor, with a dormitory, kitchenette, and lecture room on the second and third floors. The main floor parlour was the scene of many meetings of the Alumnae Association of the St. Mary's School of Nursing, founded in 1920 and still active almost eighty years later. Sr. Mary Dorothea served as the association's first honourary president, and in its early days the group served as a combination of junior auxiliary, professional association, and union, as well as alumnae. The group recorded minutes of its meetings until 1951, and in 1971, at the school's final graduation, it was the Alumnae Association who hosted the grad ball.

The association's first item of business was to select a school pin (at a cost of $3.75). They joined the

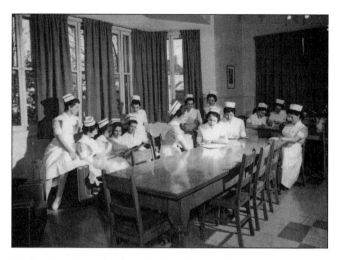

St. Mary's students in the main floor lounge of the Gibson Wing

newly formed Graduate Nurses Association of Ontario (forerunner to the RNAO) at a yearly cost of 75 cents. In 1925 the association passed a motion expressing disapproval of the twenty-four hour work day, which was the common lot of nurses at the time. In 1925 they passed a motion requesting that when doctors were arranging for private duty for General Hospital patients, that preference be given to St. Mary's graduates.

The Association put on events such as dances, card parties, etc. to raise funds for the hospital. When the school held its silver anniversary in 1933, the Alumnae Association, along with the hospital auxiliary, presided at a tea. In the 1930s, in a form of continuing education, they began to invite the hospital physicians to present lectures as part of their monthly meeting. At about the same time, the association decided against a request from the Plummer's nursing superintendent to merge the two graduate nurse associations. Finally, in a foray into the territory of the benevolent associations, in 1935 the group voted to furnish a hospital room, thus making it available for any of the members at a reduced rate ($2 per day). There is no record that this decision was ever acted upon.

Over the years, St. Mary's steadily improved its academic standards. In the early years, the full burden of lecturing fell on the town's doctors. In 1936 the school began an affiliation with Sick Children's Hospital in Toronto, and each class of students began to travel to Toronto for a twelve-week unit in pediatric nursing. This practice continued until the early 1950s when pediatrician Dr. William Robertson began to deliver lectures to the students. A similar arrangement was made with the provincial psychiatric hospitals, and in 1951 students began to travel (first to Toronto and after 1959 to North Bay) for their psychiatric training.

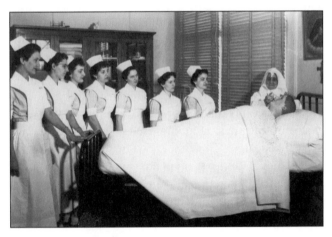

Learning patient care from Sr. John the Baptist (Susan Brennan) with the aid of "Mrs. Chase."

Through the 1930s there were unsuccessful attempts at coordination with the Plummer Hospital's school of nursing. The doctors in particular chafed at having to deliver their lectures twice. Finally in 1959 — in the first instance of formal cooperation between the two hospitals — the two schools did begin to combine some lectures. The joint lectures were delivered at the Plummer's newly opened River View Auditorium. By that time, the school had its own complement of clinical instructors.

In 1957 the school developed a professional library (similar to the doctors' medical library) and hired its own librarian. Finally, falling in step with their counterparts at other Ontario nursing schools, St. Mary's introduced the "Two plus One" course in 1966 — two years of academic training and a final year of practical training.

However, times were changing in Ontario. In 1962 the Canadian Nurses Association asked the Royal Commission on Health Services to support its stand that nursing instruction take place in institutions whose primary function was academic. By the early 1970s nursing education had moved completely from the hospitals to community colleges and universities.

Planning for the Algoma Regional School of Nursing, designed to handle the transition years from hospital control to college control, began in 1968. The school took in its first class in 1969, and St. Mary's graduated its last class in 1971. In a fitting closing of the circle, Sr. Rita Kennedy, director for thirty years at St. Mary's, became the school's first and only principal.

Through the 1950s, as class sizes grew, the hospital purchased a series of nearby private homes. The Marian Residence (at Kohler and Queen) was purchased in 1952, and the Youville Residence (directly adjacent to the hospital) in 1957. Graduates fondly remember a series of housemothers (the Misses Pim, Noble, and Henley among others) who successfully shepherded them through the training years.

School spirit and esprit de corps were always high, and St. Mary's graduates remember the camaraderie of training and the lasting friendships formed. Students lived, worked, and studied together, experiencing the pangs and pleasures of growing up away from home. Plays and concerts were prepared for parent nights, graduations, teas, and fashion shows. In 1955 Sr. Mary Emily formed a glee club to sing at graduations and masses (a task taken on by Frank Elliott in the 1960s), and a yearbook, *Fidelitas*, was begun in 1958. That year, the school's fiftieth anniversary year, was a high point with the celebrations coinciding with the hospital's sixtieth anniversary.

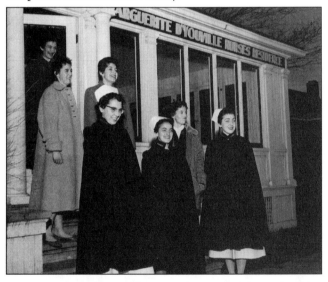

Ask any student about residence memories and they recall making friends, late leaves, room inspection, and losing privileges. Students developed lifelong bonds as they lived, learned, worked, and had fun together.

Students worked long hours. Many graduates remember making the porridge and coffee for the morning, sterilizing equipment, and sorting and rinsing laundry before it was sent from the unit. It was the good old days when all patients were bathed every day and given back rubs and mouth care every evening.

Sr. Rita Kennedy (St. Leonard) vividly remembers the 1958 June graduation ceremonies. Each graduate carried a single white rose as they filed out of the Gibson Residence and paraded down Queen Street to Precious Blood Cathedral for mass. The Knights of Columbus formed an honour guard. Following the service, the graduates filed back to the hospital for a banquet lunch and then with doctors, colleagues, church dignitaries, friends, and family looking on, the graduation exercises took place at an outdoor stage erected beside the New Pavilion (B Wing). Bishop Alexander Carter, a former chaplain, delivered the address. That evening, wearing the traditional white gowns, the graduates and their escorts attended the Gold and Diamond Ball at St. Mary's College.

The final class graduated in 1971, and then, like the spacious porches of the old hospital, St. Mary's School of Nursing was a memory. The May ceremony was held in the new Korah Collegiate auditorium in conjunction with a weekend-long reunion of all St. Mary's graduates. Thirty-eight students, including eight married students, received their caps. Dr. C.M. Eaid addressed the grads on behalf of the city's physicians. Brenda Pereplytz, winner of the General Proficiency in Nursing award, gave the valedictory address. St. Mary's instructor Leslea Anderson, who gave the keynote speech, urged the graduates to carry on the values that the school had always tried to instill in its students: "You have the foundation of nursing knowledge and skills," she said. "It's a beginning, but patients need more. We must treat them as persons first, as patients second."

More than 500 nurses graduated from St. Mary's. Most would probably agree with Ivy Reynolds as she summed up her training years fifty years later: "We had a good training," she said. The work was hard but they were happy times."

Directors of St. Mary's School of Nursing

1908	Sr. Mary Dorothea
1923	Sr. Ste. Constance
1926	Sr. Margaret Mary
1928	Sr. St. Elizabeth
1934	Sr. St. Gabriel
1935	Sr. Teresa of the Sacred Heart
1955	Sr. St. Leonard (Rita Kennedy)

Administering the Hospital

Administering the Hospital

In his address to the annual meeting in 1975, board chair James McIntyre made a perceptive comment. "It would be comforting," he said, "to predict that the present period in the hospital field will be looked on in retrospect as the difficult years. Unfortunately we may come to see them as the good old days because the pressures are not going to end."

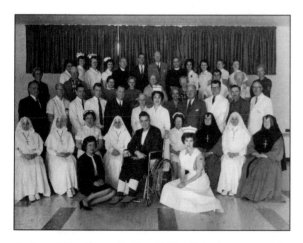

A sign of the times. By the 1960s, it took many people from many professions to provide care for one patient.

He was right. The hospital field is complex and pressure-filled and each era tends to look back at the one before it as a better and simpler time. Every administrator at the General Hospital has grappled with the problem of managing an institution that is continuously in transition, that never seems to have adequate funds and that above all else must respond to the needs of its patients.

In the earliest days job titles were simple and understandable: nurse, pharmacist, bookkeeper, domestic, gardener. Students assisted the sisters in the daily work of the hospital as well as in the care of patients. One student from the 1940s recalls that the night supervisor also looked after the switchboard in the evening, booked the next day's surgery and acted as pharmacist.

Each new decade saw changes. As physicians began to specialize and treatments became more complex, the hospital responded by hiring lay staff with very specific areas of expertise — dietitians, physiotherapists, lab technicians and pastoral care workers. Technology became more central to the hospital experience and more expensive. Workers with technical training and expertise became necessary.

A glance at some budget figures shows the

hospital's relentless growth. In 1905, eight sisters cared for about 30 patients daily. In 1934 there was a staff of 10 to 15 sisters supplemented by 13 student nurses and an operating budget of $30,790. By 1940 the budget had doubled to $68,080 and the General cared for a total of 1 800 patients annually. By 1945 the budget had doubled again to $140,700 and the number of patients also doubled, to 3,265. By 1952, with patient numbers staying almost the same at 3 924, the budget had almost quadrupled to $501,000. With a staff of 92 lay persons in addition to 20 sisters, the hospital had quietly become a sophisticated business staffed by a multitude of different professionals and support workers.

A sophisticated business needed a stable source of funds and finally in 1957 the federal Liberals passed the Hospital Insurance and Diagnostic Services Act (HIDS). Sault Ste. Marie can claim to have played a small part in the deliberations leading up to this act. Dr. Alex Sinclair recalls walking through the Plummer Hospital one day in 1952 when he met, of all people, Prime Minister Louis St. Laurent standing alone in the lobby. St. Laurent was in town for the opening of the Sault Armoury and had asked his host MP George Nixon to take him on a tour of the two hospitals so he could see for himself a community hospital and the services it provided. The HIDS was groundbreaking legislation which made hospital care universally available to all Canadians; it ushered in a two-decade period of calm and paved the way for medicare in the 1970s.

Hospital costs still continued to escalate. In 1968 the hospital's budget was $5,400,000. In 1975 it was $8,500,000 and by 1985 it had climbed to $24,800 000. A milestone was reached in 1988 when the General and Plummer in partnership acquired a CT scanner, only to be surpassed in 1998 with the purchase of an MR scanner — each one costing more

than $1,000,000. In 1997, on the eve of centennial year, the combined General/Plummer (Sault Area Hospitals) budget was $87,000,000.

But figures give only a hint of the real task. Historian Charles Rosenberg said it best — the work of every administrator, from Marie du Sauveur to Manu Malkani has been to manage this curious institution which, alone in modern society, juxtaposes high technology, bureaucracy and professionalism with the elemental human experiences of birth, death and pain.

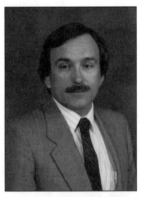

Jerry Betik was the hospital's first lay administrator.

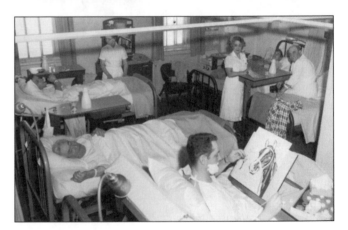

The old hospital was badly overcrowded by the time the new hospital was ready.

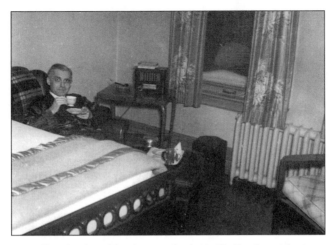

A patient in the old private unit (100 B). In the early days, hospitals were expected to encourage private patients and use the revenue from their care to subsidize non-paying patients.

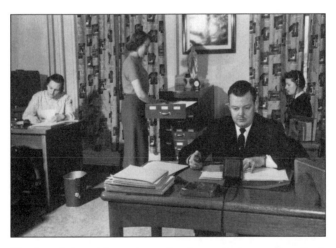

The hospital world was becoming increasingly complex. Dr. J. Gibson dictates chart notes with Medical Records staff H. Anderson and A. Desjardin.

Hospital Administrators

1898	Sr. Marie du Sauveur (Sophronie Doray)
1908	Sr. St. Jacques (Margaret Grierson)
1913	Sr. Marie de la Redemption (Helen Brennan)
1918	Sr. Marguerite Howley
1926	Sr. St. Josephat (Anna Senecal)
	— change in ownership —
1926	Sr. Mary Dorothea (Eleanor O'Driscoll)
1935	Sr. St. Elizabeth (Margaret Spooner)
1939	Sr. Mary Brigid (Mary Brigid Griffin)
1948	Sr. Mary Augustine (Patricia Redmond)
1954	Sr. Mary Dolores (Laura Anderchek)
1960	Sr. Mary Camillas (Agnes O'Callaghan)
1963	Sr. Teresa Agatha (Teresa Doyle)
1970	Sr. Shirley Crozier (Sr. St. Kevin)
1975	Sr. Mary Francis (Anita Buckley)
1985	Jerry T. Betik
1993	Manu A. Malkani

Chiefs of Staff*

1945	Dr. John H. Duncan
1947	Dr. Charles H. Greig
1972	Dr. William J. Kelly
1975	Dr. J. Pat O'Neill
1985	Dr. Bruce A.J. Skinner
1989	Dr. Ihab Kamal
1993	Dr. Bruce A.J. Skinner

* pre-1945 records unavailable

Board Chairs*

1945	J. Ryan
1949	F.L. Redden
1951	John Lang
1953	G. A. McGuire
1956	E. A. Kelly
1957	Henry Lang
1968	Dr. William Hutchinson
1970	R.B.V. Burgoyne
1975	James McIntyre
1977	Judge James Greco
1981	Bill Struk
1985	Dr. Lou Lukenda
1989	Charles Vaillancourt
1991	Rosemary O'Connor
1994	Dr. Michael Nanne
1997	Michael Mingay

* pre-1965 records are incomplete
Until 1965, the board was called the Lay Advisory Board

The Community

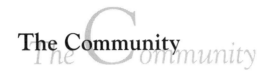

Much was owing … to the generous cooperation of the always kindly
and helpful citizens of the city and district,
to whom the Auxiliary are deeply grateful

1938 Report of the Auxiliary President

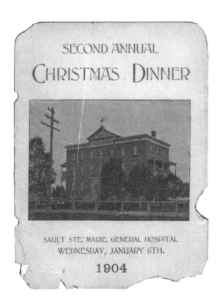

The printed menu which accompanied the Christmas
Dinner. The Committee of Management for the dinner
were: Mrs. Reid, president and Mrs. Kennedy, Durham,
Hocking, Sjostedt, Aubin, O'Boyle, Norris, C.N. Smith, S.
O'Connor, McPeak, and Miss Plummer.

Sault Ste. Marie Hospital Core Values

Sacredness of Life calls us to respect the dignity of persons and life from conception to natural death.

Hospitality
Spirituality
Vision
Justice
Sacredness of Life

The General Hospital Auxiliary

The General Hospital Auxiliary

The Ladies' Auxiliary of the General Hospital was constituted in May of 1899, just before the hospital's July opening. These women were an advance guard of the growing social awareness movement, which was taking hold in Canada. In the 20th century this would result in our comprehensive social safety-net legislation, including the Canada Health Act.

Making a go of a hospital, such a new and untried institution, was a risky proposition, and the women of the Auxiliary stepped forward to do the best they could for their neighbours and their community. On May 30, 1899, about forty women assembled at the hospital, and under the chairmanship of the indefatigable Dr. Gibson, formed the association. Mrs. W.H. (Maria) Plummer was elected president. There were four vice presidents — Mrs. O'Connor (wife of the judge), Jenny Gibson (wife of Dr. Robert), Mrs. W. O'Brien, and Mrs. Westcott. Miss Fleming was elected secretary and Mrs. Simpson, treasurer.

A constitution was prepared and published immediately, stating that the group's objective was "to co-operate with the Reverend Sisters in charge, in the work of the General Hospital, Sault Ste. Marie, in raising funds and otherwise as shall be deemed expedient." The annual membership fee was set at fifty cents (payable in advance), and meetings were scheduled to be held on the second Tuesday of each month. The constitution noted that all meetings were to begin and end with prayer. The executive committee of sixteen would be elected at each annual meeting. Many well-known Sault names appear among the Auxiliary membership: Alderdice, Aubin, Brazeau, Burden, Clergue, Desjardins, Farwell, Faulkner, Fleming, Franz, Hocking, Hussey, Lang, Lyons, McLean, McLurg, McPeak, Morin, O'Boyle, O'Connor, Plummer, Reid, Robins, Shields, Simpson, Sullivan, and Taillefer.

In the early years, the Auxiliary held a yearly charity ball, a concert, and a garden party. The group's dual roles were as fundraisers and hospital hostesses. They attacked both roles with passion, and detailed newspaper accounts chronicled their successes.

Their first project was to fundraise for operating room equipment. By the following summer, the equipment had been successfully purchased and the *Sault Express* noted that they were thanked by Dr. Gibson, who "gave the ladies a brief review of the work that was being done in the institution. In the course of his remarks the doctor stated that the operating room was now quite as well equipped as many of the best hospitals to be found in the large cities of the Dominion, a statement received with much satisfaction by the ladies."[54] The same item concludes by saying that following the meeting, "The ladies lined up in front of the building, looked their prettiest and had their photographs taken and then went home, tickled to pieces at the success of their work." Alas, no copies of these photographs remain.

The charity ball of 1900 netted $375, which the association dispersed as follows — $200 towards the laundry building then under construction (this was one fifth of the building's total cost), $25 for linens, and $80 toward the purchase of a cabinet for the operating room.

In 1902, the Auxiliary presented a July garden party and strawberry festival — a popular event taken up again eighty years later by the newly formed General Hospital Foundation.

The garden party was held on the back grounds of the newly completed hospital, with the party scene "brilliantly illuminated by arclights." It featured ice cream, strawberries and cream, cake, tea, coffee, and lemonade, along with a "beautiful flower table to supply ladies and gentlemen with fragrant bouquets." The entertainment was provided by two bands, giving "some of the best selections while the sweet voiced Rose D'Erina and her gifted and versatile husband Professor Vontom have prepared a splendid program of vocal and instrumental music."[55]

In 1914 the garden party was still being held, this time in aid of the building fund for a new hospital kitchen. For this party, the hospital's beautiful western-facing sun porches (a feature of every hospital of the era) were "artistically decorated and lighted up for the occasion." The porches would be a stage for some of the Soo's best-known singers and musicians. Several children provided displays of

dancing, and there were booths displaying various delicacies for sale.

For 1916, surely one of the poorer years, the objective was to raise funds to renovate the sun parlours. Fundraising ventures included the garden party (about $200), charity ball (about $200), and euchre party ($125). President for the year was Jenny Gibson. In 1917, with an objective of installing new flooring in the wards and semi-private rooms, the Auxiliary netted $610 from the garden party.

Each year the Auxiliary coordinated a Christmas dinner for hospital patients and each year the newspapers meticulously recorded the details of the festive event. In 1908 the *Sault Star* reported that "it is well known that the fame of the citizens' dinner to the patients during Christmastide has been spread abroad and when the time for it to be given approaches a general feeling of expectation pervades the public wards for whose especial benefit this feast is prepared." Members of the Clergue entourage must have still been in town since Miss Clergue was president of the dinner and coordinator of the various committees. "All those on the committees named have telephones and will gladly hear from intending contributors."[56]

Between thirty and forty patients were served, and the dinner was counted a brilliant success. "After dinner the bankers' good cigars gave out a fragrant perfume, good to the nostrils of the smoker. The flowers were abundant and beautiful, the color scheme in red and white; the hospital colors, being especially pleasing. Miss Lewis presented Rev. Sister Superior with a magnificent bouquet of beauty roses as a slight token of their affection, from the ladies' committee. The president, Miss Clergue, begs to thank the citizens one and all for their generosity."[57]

At the 1909 dinner, "Each patient received a bouquet with his menu card and the wards were prettily decorated with the hospital colors, red and white carnations. The menu cards were more than usually beautiful this year, being of a pale aquamarine tint with the fashionable ragged edge and decorated cover. They were tied with bow knots of white holly ribbon. Mrs. C.N. Smith always presents those lovely souvenir cards and they are much prized by all connected with the dinner. The holly ribbon to tie them is a pretty fancy of Mr. D.J. O'Brien. After the dinner came the cigars, the gift of the bankers of the Soo. Could they look in and see the cheerful smiling faces in the men's ward as they watched the rings of curling smoke, they would feel doubly repaid for their generous gift. Miss Hilda Plummer, the girl violinist of the Sault, played enchantingly on her violin after dinner. Listening to her, more than one pain-racked mortal floated softly out on the river of melody to the Island of Dreams, wherever youth and hope and love are present and where pain never comes."

The list of donors and donations is reproduced each year in the newspaper and is interesting as a record of Christmas food customs at the turn of the century and of the wide variety of exotic foods available in even an isolated northern town. The donations included: a case of oranges, four pounds of chocolates, sirloin roast, one barrel apples, two bags nuts, one box figs, a goose, three grapefruit, one barrel fish, two cans evaporated milk and five pounds of candy, three-storey fruit cake, one quart marmalade, two chickens, one quarter of lamb, twenty-five pounds of pork, four quarts cream, two bottles port wine, one bottle dandelion wine, one pineapple, a gallon of olives, bananas, a bottle of lime juice, one lemon pie, black and green tea, two gems jell, one ham and a pail of candy from Candy Kitchen. Each year the list goes on and on. Even during the years of the Great War, a bounty of food, both plain and exotic, was donated — and meticulously recorded.

By 1917 the Christmas dinner was so popular that as well as food, people were donating "sets of dishes for invalid trays," flowering plants, fern stands, six silver orange spoons, and from Miss Birdie Fitzgerald of Buckingham, Quebec (just outside Ottawa), four fancy tray cloths, most likely embroidered by Miss Fitzgerald herself.

What a treat these dinners must have been for the patients, many of whom were in hospital as much because they were poor and alone as because they were ill. In the early years of the century, the hospital was still, in many cases, a place for those who had no means of support when they were stricken with an illness.

The dinner was still being reported in 1926. That year, Christmas was celebrated with a gala celebration for the patients. There was a decorated tree on each floor, and the halls and sunrooms were trimmed with wreath and bells. Santa Claus arrived, bringing (for the men's ward) tobacco, cigars, cigarettes, matches, candies, chocolate bars, fruits and toys). The donations for the dinner reflect the increasing wealth of the city and its access to exotic goods — magazines, cut carnations, oranges and walnuts, five gallons ice cream from Model Dairy, a dozen roses (American Beauties), and a box of California grapes.

Even through the tough depression years the Auxiliary was still very active, with Sabrina Hunt and Mrs. John Alderdice serving as longtime president and treasurer. Fundraisers included bingos, tag days, and raffles. Two interesting traditions that began during the 1930s were the St. Patrick's Day fundraisers (2,000 shamrocks sold in 1939!) and the annual fruit shower. During these years, the Auxiliary was successful in purchasing a new x-ray and obstetrics table.

In the tumultuous years during and following the Second World War, the Auxiliary faded away, only to be revived in 1959 by a small group of women who had successfully organized some of the previous year's hospital Jubilee festivities. With encouragement from hospital administrator Sr. Teresa Agatha, this enthusiastic group re-founded the auxiliary. There were twenty-eight members, with the first president being Kathleen West.

Once again, the Auxiliary took on its fundraising function and added to it some direct service to patients. Under the convenorship of Jeanne Breton and Marg Souliere, they immediately outfitted a small gift shop in the sunroom on the first floor (south side) of the old hospital, selling religious and handicraft items, cigarettes, and confections and under Kathleen Lang's convenorship began to make plans for a cart to travel around to the patient bedsides. Under the supervision of Helen Slattery, they established the first Candystriper program in the northern district in 1963. Many girls (and some boys who worked as porters) got their first taste of a hospital career through candystriping, and many patients were happy to see their cheerful faces.

When the new hospital opened, the gift shop was located at the rear of the lobby, beside the switchboard. In 1972, it moved to the front of the lobby, beneath the chapel, then to the west side of the lobby in 1990, and to its present location beside the cafeteria in 1996.

The new auxiliary's first special event, a June Garden Tea held on the hospital's west lawn, was a great success. Guests entered through a flower-covered trellis and were greeted by Sr. Teresa Agatha, the president, Mrs. West, and the tea convenor, Mrs. John Ryan. Tea tables were set up on the lawn (Mrs. W.J. Kelly, Mrs. Dennis O'Sullivan, Mrs. D.A. Lalonde, Mrs. Doris Denman, Mrs. Lloyd Jenkins) and the focal points were a garden swing covered in paper flowers and a large swan filled with all sorts of cut flowers (Mrs. Harold Last, Mrs. John MacNamara). There were bazaar tables (Mrs. Robert L. Curran, Mrs. Frank Richardson, Mrs. Albert Pihlaja), a baked goods booth (Mrs. Tom Danz, Mrs. Lloyd Belec), and children were entertained in a play area complete with swings, slides, and a playpen (Mrs. Michael West). Ticket convenors were Mrs. T.A. Breton and Mrs. F. Grady. Mrs. D. Kelleher was in charge of the kitchen and pourers were Mrs. John Lang, Mrs. Fred Dawson, Mrs. J.B. Symington, Mrs. E. Spratt, Mrs. D.S. Holbrook, Mrs. F. Grady, Mrs. T.A. Breton, Mrs. W.C. Franz, Mrs. R.K. Bungeroth, and Miss Patricia Rintoul.

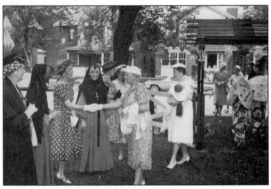

One of the first events held by the newly reorganized Ladies' Auxiliary was a June tea. This may be the 1960 tea with auxiliary president Peggy Keenan shown to the left of administrator Sr. Teresa Agatha (top photo).

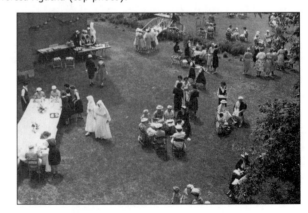

In 1961, the Auxiliary joined the Hospital Auxiliary Association of Ontario (HAAO) and began to wear their familiar pink smocks. In 1970 the General and Plummer auxiliaries jointly hosted the HAAO District Ten conference, held at the Windsor Hotel.

Over the years, the Auxiliary continued to host imaginative and successful fundraising events. Through the 1970s, the auxiliary hosted successful teas and fashion shows such as the 1973 show, convened by Nancy Allinotte with fashions from Elaine's Fashions, which netted proceeds of $2,000. In the 1980s, they sponsored hospital dinner dances. These big events were supplemented by raffles and 50/50 draws and there was always a St. Patrick's Day card party, generally held in the Officers' Mess at the Armoury.

One of the most quietly successful of the Auxiliary's fundraising programs was the Dominion Store tape program, convened by Betty Bridge. From 1973 to 1983, over $5,000,000 in cash register tapes were collected and redeemed to purchase wheelchairs and geriatric chairs, a typewriter, and refrigerator. In 1989 the Auxiliary began the sale of Nevada tickets.

For many years, the Auxiliary has been the hospital's major donor. In the 1960s their yearly donations averaged $5,000; in the 1970s, $20,000; doubling in the 1980s to $40,000, and in the 1990s to $50,000. They have furnished patient lounges, purchased sophisticated and costly medical equipment of all sorts (x-ray, ultrasound, cardiac, microscope), and funded the hospital's infant car-seat program. They have outfitted a birthing room and purchased pain pumps, fetal monitors, stretchers and NICU ventilators.

The Auxiliary established a front lobby Information Desk in 1975, a task continued by the new Volunteer Services Department. Today, most direct patient service is coordinated by Volunteer Services and the Auxiliary concentrates on its considerable fundraising

abilities. Gift shop, nevada tickets, and special draws are the Auxiliary's main source of income, with many members contributing floral arrangements, knitted baby items, and other handcrafts. Each year the Auxiliary selects its own items from the hospital's wish list and funds the purchase of those items. The process is more sophisticated than it was 100 years ago but the intent is the same. Maria Plummer and Jenny Gibson would be proud.

The Auxiliary has bestowed lifetime memberships on Jeanne Breton and Dorothy Kelleher.

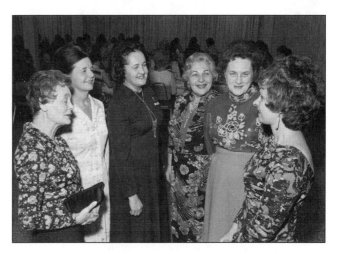

Auxiliary past presidents (left to right), Dorothy Kellher, Peggy Keenan, Kathleen West, Inez Richardson, Jeanne Breton, and Eileen Sarich gather for a photograph at a 1972 tea.

Portrait

W.H. and Maria Plummer

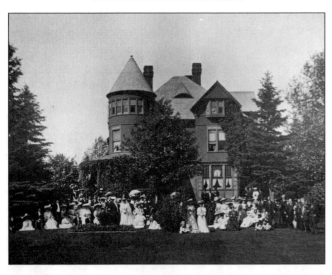

The Plummer family home "Lynnhurst" on the occasion of the marriage of their only daughter Blanche to Robert Lyon Jr. This beautiful home was donated to the city in 1920 to become the Plummer Memorial Public Hospital.

The Plummers are a perfect example of the 19th century's emerging urban middle class who worked so hard in towns all across Canada to establish and maintain hospitals.

Maria (Wiley) Plummer was born in Penetanguishine, Ontario. Her mother was a member of the Marks family, possibly a daughter of George Marks, the flamboyant merchant who successfully challenged the monopoly of the Montreal Mining Co. in the company town of Bruce Mines. Maria's cousin Jenny Marks became the wife of Dr. Robert Gibson, thereby relating by marriage the Sault's two greatest hospital champions, Gibson and Plummer. William H.

Plummer (always referred to as W.H.) was a self-made man who learned the mercantile business from the Marks brothers in Bruce Mines, probably meeting Maria there as well. They had married and come to the Sault in the early 1880s, making their home at Lynnhurst, the fabulous turreted home they built just down the street from the future General Hospital.

W.H. Plummer built up a successful trading and dry goods establishment at the corner of Queen and Pim streets, just up from the government dock. He was one of the town's greatest boosters and was part of the 1880s consortium that attempted unsuccessfully to build a power canal. Plummer was the driving force behind the committee that was finally successful in establishing the General Hospital, and he continued to take a great interest in its welfare. During a particularly strong outbreak of typhoid in 1900, the hospital ran out of bed linen when thirteen new sufferers arrived by steamer from the Helen Mine at Michipicoten. The *Chroniques* note that, knowing of the difficulties, "Plummer ran to his store and brought back as many sheets as he could carry in his arms. This excellent gentleman then assisted [the sisters] to carry the sufferers upstairs and to put them to bed, for those were days when we had no elevator."

Maria Plummer became the first president of the new hospital's Ladies' Auxiliary and was an equally tireless worker on the hospital's behalf. She had died by 1904 and was eulogised in the hospital booklet published that year:

> Her singular beauty of mind was no less remarkable than her beauty of person. Her sound sense and charming manner endeared her alike to rich and poor. She frequently brought flowers to the hospital to cheer the suffering and even during her last illness, the unselfishness which had characterized her life

remained undiminished and she ever continued to encourage the Ladies' Auxiliary to promote the interests of the hospital to the utmost.[58]

In 1920 the Plummers' lovely home, Lynnhurst, was donated to the town to house the three-year-old Royal Victoria Hospital, which was renamed the Plummer Memorial Public Hospital in their honour. The two Plummers were key players in the establishment and fortunes of both Sault hospitals. Ironically, they had both died by the opening of the second hospital, which still bears their name.

The General Hospital Foundation

The General Hospital Foundation

The General Hospital Foundation exists, according to its mission statement, "to develop, maintain and manage the funds necessary for the General Hospital to enhance or improve its services and facilities in order to continue to provide quality health care to Sault Ste. Marie and the District of Algoma." It does this by raising funds to support the hospital's capital equipment needs.

Changes in reporting requirements by the Ministry of Health led most hospitals, in the 1980s, to form foundations. Funds earned by the foundation, through fundraising and donations, were considered separate from the hospital budget and could be used to purchase specialized equipment according to varying community needs.

Letters patent were issued to the new General Hospital Foundation on April 6, 1982, with the original members of the corporation being Sr. Mary Francis, Judge James Greco, Dr. Lou Lukenda, Charles Vaillancourt, Thomas Massicotte, and Dr. Nilo Fabbro. With the addition of Derek Brisland, Len Donnelly, Sr. Jean Gray, Sr. Marguerite Hennessy, Jim McIntyre, and Henry Lang as board members, the foundation held its first meeting in June of that year. As part of that meeting the new foundation was able to gratefully acknowledge its first donation — a cheque for $50,000 from the Knights of Columbus. This was in the Knights' best tradition — they had been major donors to the campaign for the hospital's Gibson Wing almost sixty years earlier, in 1925. Along with the donation from the Knights of Columbus, the foundation began life with $600,000 from the hospital itself and $20,000 from Imperial Oil, from the dismantling of the tank "farm" located between the two hospital parking lots. The new board also took the opportunity to thank Bruce Noble and Tom Bowman, the original applicants for the letters patent, for their work and expertise in shepherding the new foundation into existence.

Some of the foundation's early projects were a cell separator ($50,000) and equipment for a new casualty room ($40,000) in Emergency. The cell separator was again a major project of the Knights of Columbus. In 1986 the Foundation contributed $100,000 toward the CAT Scan campaign.

In the early years, the foundation took on several direct fundraising projects. For several years, they hosted an art exhibition and sale with such well-known Algoma artists as Zoltan Szabo, Ken MacDougall, John Keast, Jean Burke, Fran Pond, Ken and Doug Bradford, Doug Hook, and Kathy Redmond. The Hidden Talents, a choral group of priests and the St. Michaels' Boys' Choir provided entertainment and funds in the mid-1980s. In 1987 the foundation revived an old General Hospital tradition when it hosted the first of several successful Strawberry Socials on the hospital's front lawn. Since 1990 the foundation has offered a very successful annual car draw.

Since the General's partnership with the Plummer Hospital in 1993, the two foundations have worked in concert. They undertook their first joint fundraising campaign in 1994 and are at present exploring the concept of amalgamation.

Foundation Presidents

1982	Tom Massicotte
1986	Judge James Greco
1989	Jean Lajambe
1991	Norman Candelori
1995	Rod Sonley
1997	Louise Barzan

Auxiliary Presidents

1898	Maria Plummer (wife of W.H. Plummer)
	Gibson O'Connor (wife of Judge Edward O'Connor)
	Mrs. Sullivan (wife of Charles Sullivan, merchant tailor)
	Ellen O'Boyle (wife of John O'Boyle, contractor)
	Mrs. Alderdice
	Mrs. Franz
	Mrs. John Lang
	Mrs. John Lyons
1937	Sabrina Hunt
	— reorganized in 1959 —
1959	Kathleen West
1960	Peggy Keenan
1962	Inez Richardson
1964	Kathleen West
1966	Jeanne Breton
1968	Dorothy Kelleher
1970	Eileen Sarich
1973	Marg Souliere
1975	Melva Currier
1976	Kay Clouthier
1977	Sonia Nagainis
1979	Dorothy Gabel
1981	Shirley Williams
1983	Jean Boyle
1984	Ange Parr
1985	Jean Boyle
1986	Ange Parr
1987	Jean Boyle
1988	Joyce Conway

Epilogue

100 Years of Healing, Hope, and Compassion

T.F. Chamberlain, the government inspector who in 1898, advised Sault Ste. Marie to "ask the Grey Sisters," had more wise advice for hospitals and the Ontario citizens whose taxes funded them. In his 1898 annual report, Chamberlain warned against the tendency to establish "more hospitals than the requirements of population demand, thereby dividing the work to such an extent as to cripple the efforts put forth for their proper maintenance."

"One good, well-equipped hospital," he advised, " sufficiently large to accommodate the sick of its locality, can do more and better work than two or more small hospitals, as, where duplicated in this way, the tendency is to divide the community in its philanthropic work and cause a waste of money in keeping up an extra building, staff of officers, etc. "[59]

Sault Ste. Marie was one of the first cities in Ontario to heed this advice. The partnership between the General and its sister hospital, the Plummer, was among the first in Ontario and was certainly the first between a Catholic and a non-denominational hospital.

The winds of change have blown along the St. Mary's River, past the rapids, and through the General Hospital for 100 years now and, at every gust, the hospital has trimmed its sails to stay afloat and move forward. Today, the General Hospital is utterly different from the small red-brick building the sisters first built. If the staff members of 1898 and 1998 could visit each other's workplaces, both would be incredulous at the differences they would see. But what has remained constant is the goal of expert and compassionate care in times of sickness, the goal first voiced by Dr. Robert Gibson, by W.H. and Maria Plummer, by Sr. Marie du Sauveur and Sr. Mary Dorothea, and by the community which from the beginning had generously supported the hospital.

Every staff member, every volunteer, every auxilian, every sister, every physician, every donor, if asked, "Why are you here?" would answer without hesitation, "To give good care to our patients." The theme of the General Hospital's centennial is 100 years of healing, hope, and compassion and the huge General Hospital family can be proud that, down through the years, they have given exactly that.

Appendix I
Recollections of Sr. Ste. Constance

Recollections of Sr. Ste. Constance

Sr. Ste. Constance (Clementine Gagnon) was born just outside Montreal in 1874. Her mother died when she was two and she was raised by her grandmother. She became a Sister of Charity in 1895, completed her nurse's training in 1902 at Ottawa General, and later returned to that hospital as superior and director of nurses from 1918— 1923.

From 1902 to 1908 and again from 1923 to 1926, Sr. Ste. Constance served in Sault Ste. Marie, and her memoir is a wonderful first-person description of life in the early years. Her recollection of the sorrow they felt at losing the hospital in 1926 is also one of the most moving accounts.

After leaving Sault Ste. Marie, Ste. Constance held posts at hospitals in Sudbury, Moosonee, and Ottawa. She died in 1960 at age 85.

These reminiscences (originally in French) were most likely set down in her retirement.

The Hospital at Sault Ste. Marie

In the beginning, the Sault was a very poor mission in a Protestant environment. However, what happiness we found working in this mission. The hospital is located on the beautiful and large St. Mary's River where all the passenger and freight ships dock. Directly in front is the American Sault where we could see and admire the huge lit-up factories. The gallery on the third floor was very close to the canal and from there we could see the boats arriving or bridging the 200 to 250 feet to reach Lake Superior.

Behind the house, by the river, was a magnificent vegetable garden. From the front of the house to the street was a magnificent cut lawn with several small paths and walkways where patients and staff could go for fresh air.

Beside our property, close to the river banks were two huge rocks. On Sundays, between 3:00 and 5:00 we sat between the rocks watching the arrival of passenger ships escorted by seagulls. It was quite the world on the river: sailboats, rowboats, motorboats.

If a big boat announced itself, all the small boats lined the sides of the canal to let it pass. Imagine the huge waves made by the passing of the huge ships and the small bark canoes amusing themselves riding those waves.

Now a few words about the hospital — a poor-looking house of red brick with very few conveniences; 50 beds, always occupied, not including the improvised beds when the need arose. The unexpected ill were numerous — immigrants, strangers of every language, every nationality, who arrived on the boat sick. The authorities sent them to us; we were the only hospital and the good Sister Marie du Sauveur, as they knew, refused no one.

One month after my graduation I arrived in the Sault. Here, one person must have counted for two. But there was such a good spirit of family and so much generosity that we helped each other without having to do so. Only one sister worked at night: she was responsible for three floors, answering the door and the telephone. We took a half hour break, said our prayers and started the night.

Being in charge of the operating room, I was often obliged to stay up with the patient until two in the morning. This made my nights short. If there were several patients, everyone lent a helping hand lessening the burden.

It was impossible for us to have maids; we had to do all the work ourselves. Two by two on Saturday afternoons, each on their floor, we washed the floors, stairs, kitchenettes, toilets, etc, on our knees .... After supper, the trays were cleaned for Sunday and then we tended to our personal hygiene ... haircuts with scissors for there were no clippers at the time. We went to sleep happy knowing our work was done but all the same very tired.

The population was mostly Protestant, of a good mentality and not too fanatic. We needed to deploy much zeal to gain their confidence for they had never before dealt with Sisters.

Our Mother Superior

During my stay in the Sault, I witnessed magnificent examples of charity and commitment by my Sisters. First, let's start with our dear Mother Superior, Sister Marie du Sauveur. This woman didn't know how to refuse a patient, whether Protestant or Catholic, rich or poor, infested with scabies or any other disgusting illness; she saw only Jesus in their suffering. There was nothing too good for the poor. If soup wasn't ready, she would go herself to the kitchen and cook a nice side of beef. Soon there was a good hot bowl of soup for the patient.

During her hospital rounds, if she noticed that a sister had too much to do, immediately she rolled up her sleeves and started to work; whether to wash a patient or even the bed pans. One Christmas night, we were all to go to midnight mass. At the last minute, Mother Superior said she wasn't going to mass because her legs were swollen and in pain. She sent the night nurse in her place. Upon our return at 2:00, what a surprise to see the operating room, offices, etc shining. It was a bigger surprise to see a stretcher on the floor, as well as blankets etc., What's going on? I'll tell you.

Sister Superior had received a telephone call from the company [Algoma Steel] announcing the arrival of two burn victims; both had fallen into a large bath of boiling water containing acetic and prussic acid. There was no hope of healing the two poor unfortunate victims; their skin had peeled off from their neck to their toes. So the four nurses went to work placing small two inch square bandages, soaked in oil, on all bare surfaces ... two hours of bandaging ... and the two men suffering horribly and very honourably. They were Protestant and said they regretted having disturbed us on Christmas night. Both men died six hours after having been baptized. The consolation of the Sister on duty was pouring the baptismal water which opens the doors to heaven.

Another of Sister Superior's charitable acts: there was an Indian family at the end of the city — a mother with five children, poor and miserable, whose father was dead. Sister Superior sent Dr. Gibson to get them Christmas morning. When they arrived they were given a nice bath and dressed in new clothes from head to toe. Their old clothes were burned. We knew that they would wear their new clothes all year round. At four in the afternoon, they returned home happy as kings, their arms filled with all sorts of supplies. In gratitude, the mother kissed the sisters' hands, veils and robes.

A Child with Diptheria

One festive Sunday night during break, Dr. Gibson arrived at the recreation hall asking Sister Superior if she wanted to perform an act of charity. "Certainly," she says, "if possible." "On the city limits, there is an old woman of 75 who lives in an old cabin with a small girl of five," he said. "The child has diphtheria; we have to save her." While looking at each Sister, he asked for someone to go stay at the cabin for a few days.

Sr. Superior, who didn't know how to refuse, asked who wanted to go. The first to volunteer was Sr. Ste-Désiré; very happy despite some fear of going and staying alone there in the winter. Quickly dressing in her old clothes, she left with Dr. Gibson. As Sister Ste-Désiré entered the cabin, the old Protestant woman gave her a wary look and sister's heart froze. The child was sleeping on a piece of lambskin and straw and in the cabin, Sister did not see even a chair to serve as a bed.

Before leaving, the Doctor left her the necessary remedies and later told us, "I tell you I cried when I returned home to leave Sister there and I said to my wife 'there are only nuns that can stand things like this.'" In the morning, he was the first to arrive at the cabin with a basket of supplies, dishes, etc. During the day, Sister Superior didn't forget her exiled; she sent her plenty of sweets and everyone sent her little notes. During the day, Sister Ste-Désiré kept busy cleaning the cabin, washing blankets and succeeded in making herself a proper bed where she would be able to sleep a bit. She stayed there for 15 days, healed the child and won over the old woman. What a celebration on her return. Sister Superior gave her 15 days off.

Experiences while Fundraising

Lost in the forest one day, our driver succeeded in reaching a hunter's cabin at 6 in the evening. We were frozen to the bone and our horses were exhausted. We succeeded in opening the padlock and our driver made a fire. All of a sudden, the hunter appeared — a man of six feet plus and of unusual size; he didn't seem happy to have found strangers in his cabin. The good Sister Ste-Apolline, with her usual politeness, explained our misfortunes — the cold, the hunger, our exhausted horses who travelled all day without food, etc. This dear man took pity on us; he started us off with an excellent glass of Scotch then made us supper — pork and beans, strong coffee, and brioches. After supper he went out to the fork in the road to meet a traveller who would be responsible for bringing us to our desired destination. During this time our hunter melted snow to give water to the horses. He returned saying that a hay ride was en route to the camp. We were 18 miles away from our post. The hunter settled us between two large bundles of hay and tied the horses behind the wagon where they ate their fill.

Needless to say, we were very tired upon our arrival at the camp around 2:00 in the morning. The Bourgeois went to a lot of trouble to house us. All his men were sleeping. He prepared the office with blankets, making us beds on the floor. I assure you that I didn't worry about conveniences; I threw myself on the floor, dressed, and slept. My companion however had time to find the bed hard. This camp was not our desired destination, so we went back on the road, better informed this time.

We had another experience which should have cost us our lives: we were collecting for charity at the Michipicoten mine on the upper part of Lake Superior. We went by boat from Sault Ste. Marie returning with $200 after having almost drowned in Lake Superior. There was a terrible wind storm with rain and snow; three times our boat almost capsized. One time, among others, the boat tipped so heavily on its side that a wave engulfed the boat entirely, taking everything on deck into the water. Remember Lake Superior is like the sea; the waves reach heights of 100 to 200 feet.

Needless to say, we held the rosary between our fingers. The storm lasted two hours; we were bruised everywhere having been hit so many times and pressed against the walls. The five hour trip had lasted 12 hours and everyone was sick except the two Grey Sisters who held their own. Please believe that upon our return we were bedridden for three days ... and to laugh about it afterwards ... our troubles, the discouraged faces, etc.

Typhoid Fever

What can you say about the dedication of the Sisters during the typhoid fever epidemic? Only the good Lord knows the sacrifices we made, first by giving up our own beds for the sick. Sister Supérieure went to sleep upstairs in the wash house, a sort of attic; another sister slept on a sofa in the dining hall. Four others went to sleep at the neighbour's on the other side of the street [Mrs. Smith]. At 11:00 we returned to the hospital to help the night nurse give baths and wash mouths. At 1:00 we returned to our beds, to return again to the hospital at 4:20 to bathe the patients. This lasted four weeks.

Five Frozen Sailors

After the epidemic, the dormitory needed a major clean-up: painting, washing ... Sister Supérieure had bought mattresses, pillows and blankets. When all was done ... what joy to reclaim our beds ... to lie on our two pillows and sleep. At 3:00, Dr. Gibson received a telegram from Toronto asking him to go get five sailors, probably frozen, in the Michipicoten woods in upper Lake Superior. Was it December of 1906 or 1907? There was nothing more important than going to the Sisters to ask them to prepare beds. What do you do? No beds were available except our own. The sick can't be refused. Together, without a word, we climbed to the very clean and very white dormitory, quickly replacing our mattresses with the disinfected ones. Before leaving, the Doctor asked that we have everything ready: brandy, needles, hot water. We waited for our patients all night. Not until 3:00 in the morning did we hear the bells ... three ambulances arrived.

It's almost impossible to describe the condition of the poor unfortunate sailors. They were so frozen that not one of their limbs would bend, making it impossible to undress them. They were as stiff as boards. What a day we had. For four hours, all we were able to do was give them hot brandy every 15 minutes and pour water all over their bodies to thaw their clothes and cut them away. It wasn't until midnight that this work was completed. The patients started showing faint signs of life. Everywhere their skin began peeling to the point that it was impossible to use a hypodermic needle to inject them with stimulants.

At 8:00 at night their general condition allowed us to amputate. They had gangrene of the feet, hands, ears, nose. One of them died at around 3:00 in the afternoon [J. McDonald], a young Scotsman of 22. He was fortunate to have been baptized before dying.

The other four were from Britain. At 8:00 that night, the operations began. We could not save their feet. All of them were missing a hand or an arm. Four doctors shared the work. The four patients stayed in our dormitory for five weeks and Sister Ste-Constance was their nurse. For three weeks she had not even an hour's rest between 7:00 a.m. and 11:00 p.m. Around 2:30 a.m. she woke up to give them a little comfort during the rest of the night. If there are great sacrifices to make, there are also great spiritual consolations. I thank God for that.

These men were on their first trip to Canada. Not knowing the climate, they dressed lightly. Their boat sank in Lake Superior and several sailors perished. Five made it onto the ice but as they didn't know the area, they got lost in the woods. It was only eight days later that a native government hunter found them in a hole in the snow. That day, believing they were going to die, the men had sacrificed their lives, hanging on to each other in that hole.

The Indian who found them made them a nice fire, gave them his supplies then retraced his steps to get help. Three days later, they arrived at the hospital.

Raising Money in the Alabama and Blind River Lumber Camps

It happened in the month of March in 1908. The fundraisers were Sr. Ste. Constance and Sr. Ste. Apolline, who were both on a mission for the hospital in Sault Ste. Marie. Between the years 1900 and 1910, this mission was very poor; the revenue didn't cover the expenses. Ways had to be found to raise funds to provide at least the necessities. The government only gave 15 cents a day for immigrants and as the municipality was not organized, it did not feel responsible for the poor, especially immigrants.

Sault Ste. Marie was considered a sea port since all the boats coming from England and elsewhere stopped over at this port, either to unload cargo or to take back merchandise. A large number of immigrants from the old countries traveled on these boats; a large number of them arrived sick and were sent to our hospital. Those who knew Sister Marie-du-Saveur, at that time the Mother Superior, knew that she was not one to refuse the sick because they didn't have money to pay; whether they were black or white, they were sick and had to be admitted, to be made comfortable and to be given the care they needed. So there was always a large number of immigrants — Finnish, Polish, Russian — who were all admitted for free. Many promised to come back and pay but we never saw them again. The government as well as the municipalities refused to pay, so every year a large deficit showed in the books. We had to find ways to remedy this problem. We held country fairs, raffles etc. in the summer but it wasn't enough. Therefore in the winter, funds were collected from the churches and the lumber camps: The lumber camps were the most encouraging because they brought in tidy sums of $1,500 to $1,800.

But what sacrifices on these excursions. First, the cold and all sorts of inconveniences. If we stayed with a family, we had to share the bed with the mother and her child. We would have much preferred to sleep on the floor close to the stove but the dogs would have refused to give up their spots.

Here is an experience that should have cost us our lives. One beautiful mild morning, we had decided to walk to the neighboring lumber camp two miles away, saving us two days. We were following the railway tracks because the train wasn't scheduled to pass that day so we had nothing to fear. While walking we said our rosary. The path was winding and the railway tracks snow-covered; it was as if we had been thrust between two huge mountains, the path very narrow. We had just crossed over the "footbridge" which is extremely long when suddenly a machine fast approached us. It was a snow blower. Like a bolt of lightening we each threw ourselves onto the sides of the track sinking up to our necks in the snowy void 15–20 feet deep. Each thought the other was dead. Finally, with great difficulty, I climbed out to go to the aid of my companion who wasn't able to free herself; she couldn't see a thing because her glasses were frosted. The Lord's very special protection was with us for we had no injuries except that we shook with fear until the next day.

We found the way long. We had encountered two Russians and Sister Ste. Apolline asked them if the camp was far. "Camp?" replied one of them and bent over the snow to trace with his mittened thumb the route we should follow. When he was finished he kissed our hands. We continued on our way and arrived at the exact lumber camp we were looking for, always thanking the good Lord for his protection.

It was the Alabama lumber camp in Blind River in February of 1908. It was the last stop before taking the road back to the Sault. What luck! The lumber camp was run by Mr. McGibbon; Mr. Fleming, the assistant; Mr. Faulkner, the scaler, and Mr. Fournier, the cook, the only Canadian, from the Baie des Chaleurs. There were 300 men at the camp. All of them were Protestant.

After supper we went to the lumberjacks' camp. They were sitting around the big hall, also the dormitory, lined with bunk beds, waiting for us. Seeing them sitting on the edge of their beds, their legs dangling, gave you a little chill when you entered. Soon, they put you at ease because they were polite.

We proceeded, Mr. Gibbons first, then the assistant, the two Sisters and the cook who accompanied us carrying a lantern. Each lumberjack gave his name

and the amount he wanted to give; we collected almost $400. The rounds took a good two hours because the men all had questions to ask us: our name; where we came from; what we did; how long we had been in the convent; if we were "finisher sisters." They could not understand that we would never be returning home to our families.

After the rounds, we returned to the office for the Bourgeois to write us a cheque; we never kept cash on us. The evening lasted well until 11:00 before the Bourgeois spoke about going to bed. But before going to bed, he made a suggestion that wasn't to our liking. Usually, we were given the office and the men went to sleep elsewhere. He wanted to divide the room in two with blankets and the men would stay with us. Their excuse was that it was very cold and that they had to look after the fire. Sister Ste. Appoline held her ground and the Bourgeois decided to go sleep with the other men. Finally, we were alone.

Quickly we prepared for bed. Out of regard for my precious health, Sister Ste. Appoline made me sleep at the far end of the bed; she intended to get up to make the fire ... so I said my prayers and settled in. My companion stayed seated beside the stove to finish her prayers; she always had much to say to the good Lord and favors to ask.

The account goes on to describe a terrifying night of strange noises, which the sisters attributed to the devil. More likely it was the men playing a practical joke!

I should have given a description of the office at the beginning. It was a one-room, small building, 15 by 15. In the centre was the stove made of timber with the joints held together by soil and moss. The inside walls were covered with black felt-lined paper to break the wind. In a corner, were two bunk beds made of rough boards fitted with hay and covered with gray wool blankets. In another corner the assistant's office, a counter, a desk and on the wall were fairly large shelves where the items for sale were placed: blankets, sweaters, moccasins, mittens, etc. On the other side was a table on which were found a cauldron of water, a basin, some soap and a towel. A huge lamp hung from the ceiling while mittens and toques hung on sticks to dry.

These are my fundraising experiences, Mother. I'm sorry this is not better written; maybe one of the good Sisters could rewrite it. I wouldn't mind.

Appendix II
Board of Directors and Medical Staff

BOARD OF DIRECTORS 1998

Michael Mingay, Chair
Sister Diane Carty, Vice Chair
Manu Malkani, President and Chief Executive Officer
Dr. Peter Apostle, President Medical Staff
Sam Colizza
Joyce Conway, President of Auxiliary
Sister Madeline Cooke
Nancy Cresswell
Sister Jean Gray
Mark Lajambe
Timothy Lukenda
Ron Marr
Bishop Bernard Pappin
Dr. Michael Nanne
Dr. Bruce Skinner, Chief of Staff
Rod Sonley
Evelyn Theriault
Rev. Randy Thomas
Dr. Gene Turgeon, Vice President Medical Staff

Family & Emerg. Medicine

Aleixandre, Dr. L.E.
Apostle, Dr. P. D.
Armstrong, Dr. R.D.
Avery, Dr. P.K.
Balogh, Dr. A.
Barrett, Dr. E.A.
Battel, Dr. L.A.
Beduhn, Dr. E.E.
Blois, Dr. H.
Bondar, Dr. S M.
Bragaglia, Dr. P.J.
Brooks, Dr. D. E.
Bruni, Dr. C.A.
Buehner, Dr. S.
Catania, Dr. P.
Chawla, Dr. R.
Chow, Dr. P.
Clarke, Dr. J.A.
Crookston, Dr. D.G.
Cziffer, Dr. A.
DeLuco, Dr. A.T.
Eaid, Dr. C. R. M.
Emerson, Dr. K.
Febbraro, Dr. M.A.
Febbraro, Dr. S.M.
Fera, Dr. D.J.
Fraser, Dr. R.
Fritz, Dr. D.R.
Gieni, Dr. R.M.
Grosso, Dr. W.T.
Gualazzi, Dr. D.A.
Hackett, Dr. M.A.
Hiron, Dr. P.A.
Hogg-Kuntz, Dr. E.
Hoogeveen, Dr. P.
Ianni, Dr. F. A.

Jablanczy, Dr. A.
Keating, Dr. M.V.
Kelly, Dr. M.J.A
Kobelka, Dr. C.
Kuntz, Dr. M.P.
Lane, Dr. J.C.
Lang, Dr. S. R.
Leahy, Dr. M.
Lee, Dr. A.F.
Luus, Dr. G.
Macmichael, Dr. G.K.
Maione, Dr. P.F.
Maloney, Dr. R.J.
Marrack, Dr. J.E.
McLean, Dr. A.D.
McLeod, Dr. J.
Mogharrabi, Dr. M.
Naigamwalla, Dr. J.B.
O'Brien, Dr. L.J.
Pearson, Dr. J.C.
Poitevin, Dr. D.G.
Quon, Dr. D. A.
Rilett, Dr. J.
Roedde, Dr. S.
Rossi, Dr. C.M.
Schwarz, Dr. P.
Shamess, Dr. B.A.
Smith, Dr. N.A.
Turgeon, Dr. E.W.T
Vilcini, Dr. M.M.
Wacker, Dr. K.P.
Waymouth, Dr. W.E.
White, Dr. E.
Wytsma, Dr. R.

Family Med. — Courtesy

* Hackett, Dr. A.A.

* Kirby, Dr. E.
* Sullivan, Dr. W.E.

Diagnostic Imaging

D'Ovidio, Dr. R.G.
* McNair, Dr. D.J.
Stenning, Dr. D.
Scarff, Dr. M.A.

Anaesthesia

* Brereton, Dr. W.
Hadley, Dr. L.D.
Norris, Dr. D.
Owen, Dr. J.E.L.
Taylor, Dr. M.J.

Ophthalmology

Bariciak, Dr. M.D.
Beauchene, Dr. R.
Golesic, Dr. G.F.
Mitchell, Dr. B.J.
Sharp, Dr. D. C.
* Stevenson, Dr. R.F.

Obstetrics/Gynaecology

Amimi, Dr. M.
Fam. Dr. P.
Hergott, Dr. P.A.
Hutton, Dr. W.F.
* Lalouette, Dr. J.
* Miller, Dr. N.E.
Olupona, Dr. S.M.
Willett, Dr. J.A.
Zehr, Dr. P.

Psychiatry

* Bourdeau, Dr. D.
* Byers, Dr. J.
* Carr, Dr. A.
* Chaimowitz, Dr. G.
* Chisvin, Dr. M.
* Cook, Dr. P.
* de Groot, Dr. J.
* Darby, Dr. C.
* Ferencz, Dr. J.
* Gort, Dr. G.
* Hodges, Dr. B.
* Karunaratne, Dr. K.
* Letourneau, Dr. G.
Leung, Dr. H.H.
* Lofchy, Dr. J.
* Malcolmson, Dr. S.
* Persad, Dr. E.
Pistor, Dr. L.
Tang, D.
* Ulzen, Dr. T.
* Webb, Dr. S.

Pathology

Chawla, Dr. S.
Mozarowski, Dr. P.T.
O'Hara, Dr. K.E.
Rasaiah, Dr. R.

Internal Medecine

Bignell, Dr. D.C.
* Bowen, Dr. J.
* Bruni, Dr. J.
Ciaschini, Dr. P.
Conly, Dr. D.B.
Farah, Dr. S.S.

Gieni, Dr. J.L.
Gould, Dr. D.H.
Gupta, Dr. I.P.
Jenkins, Dr. C.O.
* Karsan, Dr. F.
* Kirshen, Dr. A.J.
Lee, Dr. H.N.
* Leung, Dr. F.Y.K
Mathew, Dr. M.T.
* Muirhead, Dr. N.
* Nolan, Dr. W.T.
* Patterson, Dr. C.
Robertson, Dr. J.W.
* Secord, Dr. G.V.
Skinner, Dr. B.A.J.
Spadafora, Dr. S.
Tawfik, Dr. N.H.
Walde, Dr. P.L.D.
West, Dr. M.H.

Surgery

Armstrong, Dr. J.K.
** Baar, Dr. F.
Best, Dr. T.
Bharadwaj, Dr. V.K.
Casses, Dr. A.
Fratesi, Dr. S.J.
Fyfe, Dr. P.R.
Jacqmin, Dr. M.
Kolodziejczyk, Dr. K.
* Lalonde, Dr. A.H.
Mathur, Dr. V.K.
McAllister, Dr. T.
Mohamed, Dr. J.K.
Mossing, Dr. M.S.
O'Neill, Dr. J.P.
Sewards, Dr. H.F.G.

** Sinclair, Dr. A.B.
Taylor, Dr. R. D.
Woolner, Dr. D.S.

Paediatrics

Burrows, Dr. D.R.
Chen, Dr. C.P.
Lam, Dr. K.L.
*Lyttle, Dr. B.
Muhlstein, Dr. T.R.
* Robertson, Dr. W.J.
Zufelt, Dr. K.

* Courtesy Staff
** Honourary Staff

Bibliography

Sault Ste. Marie

Bothwell, Robert. *A Short History of Ontario.* Edmonton: Hurtig Publishers, 1986.

Burtch, Linda. *Great Lakes Power: 75 Years of Continuous Progress.* Sault Ste. Marie: n.p., 1991.

Capp, Edward H. *The Story of Baw-a-ting, Being the Annals of Sault Sainte Marie.* Sault Ste. Marie: Sault Star Printers, 1904.

Heath, Frances M. *Sault Ste. Marie: City by the Rapids, An Illustrated History.* Burlington: Windsor Publications, 1988.

MacDowell, Laurel Sefton. "New Ontario: The North Before and After 1884." *Loyal She Remains: A Pictorial History of Ontario.* Toronto: United Empire Loyalists' Association of Canada, 1984.

MacKay, Donald. *The Lumberjacks.* Toronto: McGraw-Hill Ryerson, 1978.

McDowall, Duncan. *Steel at the Sault: Francis H. Clergue, Sir James Dunn, and the Algoma Steel Corporation 1901–1956.* Toronto: University of Toronto Press, 1984.

Mount, Graeme S., John Abbott, and Michael J. Mulloy. *The Border at Sault Ste. Marie.* Toronto: Dundurn Press, 1995.

Nock, O.S. *Algoma Central Railway.* London: A & C Black, 1975.

Patterns of the Past: Interpreting Ontario's History. Toronto: Dundurn Press, 1988.

Health and Medicine

Agnew, G. Harvey. *Canadian Hospitals 1920–1970: A Dramatic Half-Century.* Toronto: University of Toronto Press, 1974.

Annual Report of the Inspector of Prisons and Public Charities upon the Hospitals and Charities, Etc. of the Province of Ontario. Toronto: L.K. Cameron, 1898–1909.

Dictionary of Canadian Biography. Toronto: University Press, 1969.

Connor, Ralph. *The Doctor: A Tale of the Rockies.* Toronto: Westminister Co., 1906.

Gagan, David. "For Patients of Moderate Means: The Transformation of Ontario's Public General Hospitals, 1880–1950." *Canadian Historical Review.* 70, 1989. 151–179.

The Hospitals of Ontario. Toronto: Herbert H. Ball, 1934.

Lessard, Renald. *Health Care in Canada During the Seventeenth and Eighteenth Centuries.* Ottawa: Canadian Museum of Civilization, 1991.

MacDermot, H.E. *One Hundred Years of Medicine in Canada 1867–1967.* Toronto: McClelland and Stewart, 1988.

McPherson, Kathryn. *Bedside Matters: The Transformation of Canadian Nursing, 1900–1990.* Ottawa: Oxford University Press, 1996.

Mitchinson, Wendy and Janice Dickin McGinnis. *Essays in the History of Canadian Medicine.* Toronto: McClelland and Stewart, 1988.

Roland, C.G., ed. *Health, Disease and Medicine: Essays in Canadian History.* Toronto: Hannah Institute for the History of Medicine, 1984.

Rosenberg, Charles E. *The Care of Strangers: The Rise of America's Hospital System.* New York: Basic Books, 1987.

Ross, Mary A. "Typhoid Fever Mortality in Ontario, 1880–1931." *Canadian Public Health Journal* 26: 73–84. 1935.

Shortt, S.E.D. *The Canadian Hospital in the 19th Century: An Historiographic Lament.* Journal of Canadian Studies. 18:4, 1983–84. p. 3–14.

Vayda, Eugene and Raisa B. Deber. "The Canadian Health-Care System: A Developmental Overview." *Candian Health Care and the State: A Century of Evolution.* Montreal: McGill-Queen's University Press, 1992.

Grey Sisters

Cellard, Andre and Gerald Pelletier. *Faithful to a Mission: Fifty Years with the Catholic Health Association of Canada.* Ottawa: Catholic Health Association of Canada, 1990.

Courneene, Sr. Erma. *Foundation of the Grey Sisters of the Immaculate Conception.* Pembroke: n.p., 1977.

The Grey Nuns of the Cross (Sisters of Charity of Ottawa) Evolution of the Institute 1876–1967. Ottawa: n.p., 1989.

Keefe, Sr. Thomas Aquinas. *The Congregation of the Grey Nuns (1737–1910).* Washington, D.C.: Catholic University of America, 1942.

King, Dennis. *The Grey Nuns and the Red River Settlement.* Agincourt: The Book Society of Canada. 1980.

McGuire, Sr. Rita. *Marguerite d'Youville: A Pioneer for our Times.* Ottawa: Novalis, 1982.

Mitchell, Estelle. *The Spiritual Portrait of Saint Marguerite d'Youville.* Montreal: Palm Publisher, 1965.

Souvenirs Intimes de notre Famille Religieuse. Ottawa: Soeurs Grises de la Croix, n.d.

General Hospital

Carriere, Marylyn R., et al. A Health Service Partnership in Sault Ste. Marie, Ontario. *Strategic Alliances In Health Care.* Ottawa: Candian College of Health Services Executives, 1996.

Gimby, W.E. *A History of the Medical Profession.* Sault Ste. Marie: Sault Star Printers, 1922.

McL., M.C. *Outline of the History and Management of the General Hospital.* Sault Ste. Marie: Sault Star Printers, [1906].

O'Donnell, William. *The Worst Epidemic Ever: Spanish Influenza 1918.* Unpublished manuscript.

Plummer, J.O. *Canadian Pioneers: History of the Plummer Family.* Privately Published, n.d.

Diaries
Chroniques de l'Hopital General de Sault-Ste-Marie 1896–1926.
Annals of the General Hospital, Sault Ste. Marie 1926–1954.
Personal reminiscences of four early Sisters (including Sr. Ste. Constance)

Minutes
General Hospital Admissions Register 1923–1930.
General Hospital Board of Directors 1965–1998.
General Hospital Medical Board 1921–1947.
General Hospital Nurses' Alumnae Association 1920–1951.
General Hospital Operation Register 1920–1923.
General Hospital Senior Auxiliary 1937–1939.
Sault Ste. Marie Board of Health 1895–1900.
Sault Ste. Marie Medical Society 1925–1939.
Sault Ste. Marie Town Council 1896–1899.

Miscellaneous material from archival collections held by the Province of Ontario (RG 10-54 and RG 63, Series A-7), Sisters of Charity of Ottawa (including a collection of 47 letters relating to the founding of the General Hospital to 1926 and inventory lisitings relating to the 1926 change of ownership) and the Grey Sisters of the Immaculate Conception.

Newspapers
Algoma Pioneer, Northern Ontario Record, Sault Express, Sault Star.

Pamphlets
Algoma Steel Appeals to Friends for Aid in Extending Hospital Facilities at Sault Ste. Marie (1953).
Diamond Jubilee: General Hospital 1898–1958 (1958).
The Doors that Never Close. (1961)
Let Us Lift the Burden from the Sault Ste. Marie General Hospital. (1912)

Endnotes

1. McDowall p. 29
2. *Sault Express.* June 10, 1899.
3. McDowell p.30
4. letter from F. Clergue to Dr. R. Gibson. Jan 1900.
5. *Sault Express.* July 27, 1900.
6. letter from Marie du Sauveur to Mere Kirby. August 12, 1900.
7. Gagan p.153
8. *The Hospitals of Ontario* p. 4
9. Rosenberg p.149
10. Connor p.68
11. Connor p.68
12. Courneene p. 14
13. *Chroniques* p.8
14. *Sault Star.* April 25, 1996.
15. Minutes [Sault Ste. Marie Town Council]. Dec. 21, 1896.
16. *Sault Star.* Aug. 6, 1918.
17. *A History of the Medical Profession*
18. letter from Dr. R. Gibson to Sr. St. Cyprien. June 29, 1897.
19. letter from Sr. St. Raphael to Mere Demers. June 30, 1897.
20. letter from Fr. J.A. Primeau to Mere Demers. July 20, 1897.
21. letter from Dr. R.Gibson to Mere Kirby. May, 1898.
22. letter from James Thomson to Fr. Primeau. May 31, 1898.
23. letter from Dr. R. Gibson to Mere Kirby. Aug. 4, 1898.
24. letter from Fr. J.A. Primeau to Mere Kirby. n.d.
25. *Sault Express.* Sept. 23, 1898.
26. *Chroniques.* p. 10, Sept. 28, 1899.
27. *Outline of the History and Management of the General Hospital* p. 11-12.
28. *Sault Star.* Sept. 11, 1902.
29. *Sault Star.* June 11, 1908.
30. ibid
31. *Algoma Pioneer.* June 12, 1914.
32. *Sault Star.* ? 1920.
33. letter from Mere Albert to J. Hussey. Dec. 13, 1923.
34. *Sault Star.* Feb. 17, 1925.
35. *Sault Star.* Oct. 18, 1918.
36. *Chroniques.* Oct. 1918. p.51
37. letter from Senior Auxiliary to Sr. St. Josaphat. Aug. 10, 1926.
38. letter from Bishop's House North Bay to Sr. Ste. Constance. ? 1926.
39. *Annals.* p. 1
40. ibid p. 3
41. ibid p. 4
42. ibid p.
43. ibid
44. ibid
45. ibid
46. ibid
47. speech by Minister of Health Ruth Grier to 1993 Plummer/General Annual Meeting.
48. Medical Staff Minutes. 1901.
49. ibid
50. ibid
51. ibid
52. *Sault Star.* June 18, 1958.
53. *Sault Star.* n.d.
54. *Sault Express.* July 27, 1900.
55. *Sault Express.* July 7, 1902.
56. *Sault Star.* Jan. 9, 1908.
57. *Sault Star.* Jan. 16, 1908.
58. *Outline of the History and Management* p.28
59. Report of the Inspector 1898. p.10

Index

Italics — Illustration or caption reference

Greco, Dr. B., 80
Greco, Dr. E.J.M., *77, 80*
Greco, James, 91, 102, 104
Greig, Dr. Charles H., 63, *77, 79, 90*
Grey Nuns, 14, 28
Grey Sisters, 25, 28
Grey Sisters of the Cross (Ottawa), 26, 29, 30, 31, 43, 54, 57, 58
Grey Sisters of the Immaculate Conception, 31, *31*, 32, 57, 58, 67, 73
Grier, Ruth, 73

Halton, H.R., quoted, 49-50
Hamilton, Dr. Benson, 58, 78
Hawke, John, *28*
Heath, Dr. T.R., *77*
Helidore, Sr., 48
Hennessy, Sr. Marguerite, *33*, 72, 102
Hocking, Mrs., *93*
Holbrook, Mrs. D.S., 98
Holbrook, David S., 66
Hollingsworth, Lynn, 65
Holt, Sr. Margaret, *33*
Hook, Doug, 103
Hospitals, history 1870-1920, 20-22, in New France, 25
Howley, Sr. Marguerite, 90
Hunt, Sabrina, 97, 105
Hunter, George A., 38
Hussey, J.A., 52, 54
Hutchinson, Dr. William, 68, 79, 91

Ihab Kamal, Dr., 90
Imperial Order Daughters of the Empire, 56
Indians, 13, 26, 111
Infectious diseases, 22, 51, 109; *See also* Flu epidemic, Typhoid
Jannison & Scott, 66

Jenkins, Mrs. Lloyd, 98
Jesuits, 13, 26, 44, 48, 51
John the Baptist, Sr., 84
Johnston, Dr. Hugh W., 78, *80*
Johnston, Dr. J., *77*
Jones, Col. C.H.L., 54

Keast, John, 102
Keenan, Peggy, *68*, 98, 105
Kehoe, J.J., 18, 38, 45
Kehoe, Mildred, 82
Keith, Dr. John P., 58, 78
Kelleher, Mrs. Dorothy, 98, 99, 105
Kelly, E.A., 91
Kelly, Mrs. W.J., 98
Kelly, Dr. William J., *79*, 80, 90
Kennedy, Mrs., *93*
Kennedy, Sr. Rita, 69, 84, 85, 86
Kirby, Mère Dorothy, 30, 44, 45, 48, 51, 64
Knights of Columbus, 56, 85, 102

La Vérendrye, Pierre de, 14, 15
Ladies' Auxiliary, 48, 50, 52, 53, 57, 63, 68, 71, 93-99, 100-101
Lagrave, Sr., 14
Lajambe, Jean, 104
Lajemmerais, Christophe de, 14, 15, 27
Lalonde, Dr. A., 80
Lalonde, Mrs. D.A., 98
Lamarche, Fr., 48
Lane, Dr. Robert T., 58, 78
Lang, Henry, *68*, 68, 70, 91, 102
Lang, John, 91
Lang, Kathleen (Mrs. John), 98, 105
Lang, Robert, 48
Last, Mrs. Harold, 98
Lavigne, Veronica, *75*
Leahy, Dr. W.H., 58, 78, *80*

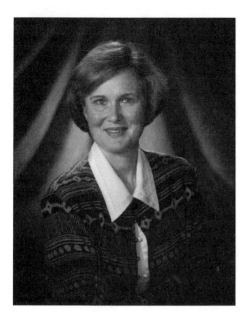

Elizabeth Iles has degrees in history from Queen's University and library science from the University of Toronto. She is the patient representative and Community Relations Officer for Sault Area Hospitals, of which the Sault Ste. Marie Hospital is a partner.